Pediatric Trauma

Proceedings of the Third National Conference

Arnold G. Coran, M.D.

Professor of Surgery
Head, Section of Pediatric Surgery
University of Michigan Medical School
Surgeon-in-Chief
C.S. Mott Children's Hospital
Ann Arbor, Michigan

Burton H. Harris, M.D.

The Orvar Swenson Professor of Pediatric Surgery
Tufts University School of Medicine
Chief of Pediatric Surgery
New England Medical Center
Director, Kiwanis Pediatric Trauma Institute
Boston, Massachusetts

With 26 Contributors

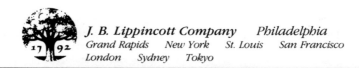

J. B. Lippincott Company   *Philadelphia*
Grand Rapids   New York   St. Louis   San Francisco
London   Sydney   Tokyo

Acquistions Editor: Lisa McAllister
Project Coordinator: Lori J. Bainbridge
Designer: Anne O'Donnell
Production Coordinator: Ruttle, Shaw & Wetherill, Inc.
Compositor: David Seham Associates Inc.
Printer/Binder: R. R. Donnelley & Sons

6   5   4   3   2   1

Library of Congress Cataloging-in-Publication Data
Pediatric trauma : proceedings of the third national conference / [edited by] Arnold G. Coran, Burton H. Harris.
       p.   cm.
       Proceedings of the Third National Conference on Pediatric Trauma,
   held in Ann Arbor, Mich., Sept. 20–23, 1989.
       ISBN 0-397-51108-6 : $45.00 (est.)
       1. Children—Wounds and injuries—Congresses.   I. Coran, Arnold
   G., 1938– .   II. Harris, Burton H.   III. National Conference on Pediatric Trauma (3rd : 1989 : Ann Arbor, Mich.)
       [DNLM: 1. Wounds and Injuries—in infancy & childhood—congresses.
   WO 700 P3714 1989]
   RD93.5.C4P46 1990
   617.1—dc20
   DNLM/DLC
   for Library of Congress   89-13740
                                                                                                                  CIP

CONTRIBUTORS

Harry Linne Anderson III, M.D.
Resident in Surgery
University of Michigan Hospitals
Ann Arbor, Michigan

Robert H. Bartlett, M.D.
Professor of Surgery
University of Michigan Medical Center
Ann Arbor, Michigan

**David H. Bass, MMed (Surg),
  FRCS (SA)**
Consultant Surgeon, University of Cape
  Town, South Africa
Specialist Surgeon and Head of
  Trauma Unit
Red Cross War Memorial Children's
  Hospital
Cape Town, Republic of South Africa

Cathy A. Burnweit, M.D.
Chief Resident in Pediatric Surgery
Hospital for Sick Children
Toronto, Ontario

Michael G. Caty, M.D.
Resident in Surgery
Department of Surgery
University of Michigan Medical School
Ann Arbor, Michigan

Arnold G. Coran, M.D.
Professor of Surgery
Head, Section of Pediatric Surgery
University of Michigan Medical School
Surgeon-in-Chief
C.S. Mott Children's Hospital
Ann Arbor, Michigan

**Sidney Cywes, MMed (Surg),
  FACS, FRCS (Eng)**
Charles F M Saint Professor of
  Paediatric Surgery
University of Cape Town
Chief Surgeon
Red Cross War Memorial Children's
  Hospital
Cape Town, Republic of South Africa

Martin Eichelberger, M.D.
Professor of Surgery and Pediatrics
George Washington University School
  of Medicine
Director of Emergency Trauma Service
Children's National Medical Center
Washington, District of Columbia

Robert M. Filler, M.D.
Surgeon-in-Chief
Hospital for Sick Children
Toronto, Ontario

Hans P. Friedl, M.D.
Postdoctoral Fellow
Department of Pathology
University of Michigan Medical
  School
Ann Arbor, Michigan

J. Alex Haller, Jr., M.D.
The Robert Garrett Professor of
    Pediatric Surgery
Professor of Pediatrics
Professor of Emergency Medicine
The Johns Hopkins University School
    of Medicine
Children's Surgeon-in-Charge
The Johns Hopkins Hospital
Baltimore, Maryland

Burton H. Harris, M.D.
The Orvar Swenson Professor of
    Pediatric Surgery
Tufts University School of Medicine
Chief of Pediatric Surgery
New England Medical Center
Director, Kiwanis Pediatric Trauma
    Institute
Boston, Massachusetts

Shelley M. Kibel, MB ChB, DCH (SA)
Medical Officer and Researcher
Department of Paediatric Surgery
University of Cape Town
Medical Officer and Researcher
Child Safety Centre
Red Cross War Memorial Children's
    Hospital
Cape Town, Republic of South Africa

Julie A. Long, M.D.
Assistant Professor of Surgery
Wayne State University
Director of Trauma
Children's Hospital of Michigan
Detroit, Michigan

Keith T. Oldham, M.D.
Associate Professor of Surgery
Section of Pediatric Surgery
University of Michigan Medical School
Attending Surgeon
C.S. Mott Children's Hospital
University of Michigan
Ann Arbor, Michigan

James A. O'Neill, Jr., M.D.
The C. Everett Koop Professor of
    Pediatric Surgery
University of Pennsylvania School of
    Medicine
Surgeon-in-Chief
The Children's Hospital of
    Philadelphia
Philadelphia, Pennsylvania

Arvin I. Philipart, M.D.
Professor of Surgery
Wayne State University School of
    Medicine
Chief of Pediatric General Surgery and
    Chairman of Surgical Services
Children's Hospital of Michigan
Detroit, Michigan

Max L. Ramenofsky, M.D.
Professor of Surgery and Pediatrics
University of Pittsburgh
School of Medicine
Director, Benedum Pediatric Trauma
    Program
Children's Hospital of Pittsburgh
Pittsburgh, Pennsylvania

G. Tom Shires III, M.D.
Assistant Professor of Surgery
Cornell University Medical College
Assistant Attending Surgeon
New York Hospital
New York, New York

Thomas C. Shope, M.D.
Associate Professor of Pediatrics
University of Michigan Medical School
Director, Pediatric Infectious Disease
C.S. Mott Children's Hospital
Ann Arbor, Michigan

Gerd O. Till, M.D.
Associate Professor
University of Michigan Medical School
Department of Pathology
Ann Arbor, Michigan

Peter A. Ward, M.D.
Professor and Chairman
Department of Pathology
University of Michigan Medical
  School
Ann Arbor, Michigan

Kathleen Weber, M.A.
Director, Child Passenger Protection
  Research Program
Department of Surgery, Section of
  Pediatric Surgery
University of Michigan Medical School
Ann Arbor, Michigan

John R. Wesley, M.D.
Associate Professor of Surgery
University of Michigan Medical School
Attending Surgeon
C.S. Mott Children's Hospital
Ann Arbor, Michigan

Douglas W. Wilmore, M.D.
Frank Sawyer Professor of Surgery
Harvard Medical School
Clinical Director of Nutrition Support
Brigham and Women's Hospital
Boston, Massachusetts

George D. Zuidema, M.D., A.B.
Vice Provost for Medical Affairs
Professor of Surgery
University of Michigan Hospitals
Ann Arbor, Michigan

PREFACE

This book is a compilation of the major lectures given at the Third National Conference on Pediatric Trauma in Ann Arbor, Michigan, on September 20 to 23, 1989. The authors of these chapters have presented the latest information available in their areas of expertise. This series of lectures is not a comprehensive review of the entire field of pediatric trauma but rather highlights the major clinical and experimental advances. We hope this book will act as a stimulus for future clinical and laboratory research in this rapidly growing field of pediatric care.

Arnold G. Coran, M.D.
Burton H. Harris, M.D.

CONTENTS

Pediatric Trauma

Proceedings of the Third National Conference

CHAPTER 1

Toward a Comprehensive Emergency Medical System for Children

J. Alex Haller, Jr.

S ystems management of life-threatening injuries in children and adults is now accepted in the United States and Canada as state of the art care for trauma victims. A few regional trauma systems for adults have had several decades of experience and have served recently as models for inclusion of pediatric trauma.[1] In certain areas, notably Pennsylvania, an emergency medical system with fully integrated adult and children's components has come into being. The National Pediatric Trauma Registry, which includes more than 12,000 children, is indicative of the significant problem of trauma in this age group and offers a base for statistical analysis of injury severity and long-term rehabilitation needs.[2]

Since 1985, several projects under federally funded state demonstration grants for pediatric emergency medical services have attempted to establish guidelines for patient care and to suggest methods for ongoing monitoring of these systems' effectiveness, surveillance of quality, and review of patient outcome.

A statewide, designated pediatric trauma center for Maryland, located in The Johns Hopkins Children's Center, has functioned for 12 years.[3] Data are now available to allow some objective evaluation of the effectiveness and impact of this regional pediatric trauma program.

The level of compliance within Maryland's regionalized pediatric trauma system from 1979 to 1986 was examined recently, using data recorded routinely on all discharges from 58 acute care hospitals in the Maryland.[4] Compliance with regionalization was measured by examining the proportion of patients within each category of injury severity scores (ISS) who were treated at each of three levels of care (statewide pediatric trauma center [SPTC], regional trauma center [RTC], and community hospital [COHO]) and the proportion of in-hospital deaths that occurred at each level of care. During this 8-year period, 30,214 children under 13 years were discharged from a Maryland hospital with the principal diagnosis of trauma. The proportion of patients treated at a SPTC or RTC increased from 32%

in 1979 to 42% in 1986. In the most severely injured group (ISS > 12) the proportion of patients treated at a SPTC increased from 28% to 36%. Overall, 90% of the 174 in-hospital deaths during the study period occurred in designated trauma centers. The percent treatment at SPTC, RTC, and non-RTC for each ISS group for 1986 is presented in Table 1-1 (n = 2937).

The relationship between ISS and level of care indicates good overall compliance with the system; as severity of trauma increased, the child was more likely to be treated at a higher level of care. The younger the child, the more likely the patient was to be admitted to the SPTC. Assessing and monitoring compliance with regionalization is essential in systems management and in evaluation of pediatric trauma care.

The systems approach to trauma management makes it possible to divide a region by geographic area or population composition. Maryland is divided into five EMS regions, based upon geographic and population differences. This allows for statistical evaluation of differences in types of injury (e.g., rural or mountainous areas versus densely populated metropolitan areas).

Several components are intrinsic to such a program. First, a two-way radio communication system between a hospital and emergency medical technicians at the scene of an emergency that will allow for communication with physicians, identification of medical specialists in nearby hospitals, and thus determine the destination of a child patient.

Second, a dependable transport system, preferably tax-supported, which may include several modalities. In Maryland, these components include radio-controlled police helicopter transport, which is initiated through an emergency medical relay center. Transportation to the appropriate specialty facility is arranged through the relay center for each case at the scene. In metropolitan areas of the system, ground transport is by specially equipped, fire-department-staffed ambulances, which operate under the same systems control and communication.

Third, emergency medical technicians must receive specialized training in the care of newborn infants and children from pediatric specialists such as neonatologists, pediatric surgeons, pediatric emergency physicians, and anesthesiologists. Technicians are then qualified to begin IV treatment of small infants, including intraosseous infusions, and to intubate babies and young children. Such training must be a part of the ongoing training program for emergency medical technicians within the regional system. These training programs must be carefully monitored and the technicians must be retested and retrained at appropriate intervals.

Table 1-1.

Level of Care	ISS 1–4	ISS 5–8	ISS 9–12	ISS > 12
SPTC	10%	16%	21%	37%
RTC	24%	25%	30%	36%
COHO	66%	59%	49%	27%

Fourth, designated pediatric intensive care units (ICUs) must be centralized within such a system. Within such ICUs, the patient stations must be equipped with multiple-channel monitoring equipment and ventilators, and staffed for immediate detection of cardiopulmonary arrest, for resuscitation, and for continuing post-trauma management. A small, dedicated on-site blood gas laboratory will provide immediate blood gas determination necessary for the moment-to-moment management of these unstable patients.

Fifth, an intermediate care unit is an important component of such a system. It decreases congestion in the pediatric ICU and provides "stepdown" management and continuing care while allowing more family and primary physician input.

Sixth, a dedicated pediatric rehabilitation unit, under the direction of pediatric physiatrists, neurologists, and other pediatric behavior and learning specialists, provides important support for the eventual recovery of the child trauma patient.

Finally, as asserted by the recent Ross Conference on Emergency Medical Services for Children,[5] the establishment of designated pediatric trauma centers is a natural step toward increasing systems management of life-threatening illnesses as well as injuries. As shown in Figure 1-1, an integrated system emphasizes the close interdependence of primary-care pediatricians, pediatric surgeons, emergency medicine physicians, and critical-care pediatricians in the sequential resuscitation and total management of severely ill and injured children. Within this system, emergency-care nurse specialists work closely with physicians and complete the dedicated and committed basic emergency medical team.

The recently reorganized standing Committee on Emergency Medical Services for Children of the American Academy of Pediatrics, which is composed of pediatricians, emergency physicians, and pediatric surgeons, has been charged with the responsibility of developing national standards of emergency care for children, including both life-threatening illnesses and serious injuries.

Currently, access to such EMSC systems is variable, and a strong educational effort by pediatric health-care providers will be necessary to facilitate entry into the EMSC system. Entry may occur directly from the field by means of paramedics, (e.g., with trauma), by parent transport (e.g., with high fever or seizures), or by primary-care pediatricians (e.g., family physicians) from their offices directly to the regional center or more commonly to "emergency departments appropriate for pediatric care," called EDAPs by Seidel and associates.[6] The whole system is integrated by central EMSC communication, and alarm and transport is controlled on-line by dedicated, experienced pediatric emergency physicians. The major challenge remains of establishing criteria for early detection of childhood illnesses that may rapidly become life-threatening, so that these children can enter the appropriate component of the system before death is impending.

With further integration of such emergency medical services for children and close cooperation among pediatric emergency physicians and pediatric surgeons, such systems management offers an important opportunity to extend modern pediatric critical care to children in the home, in the field, and during transport to designated centers for emergency medical care.

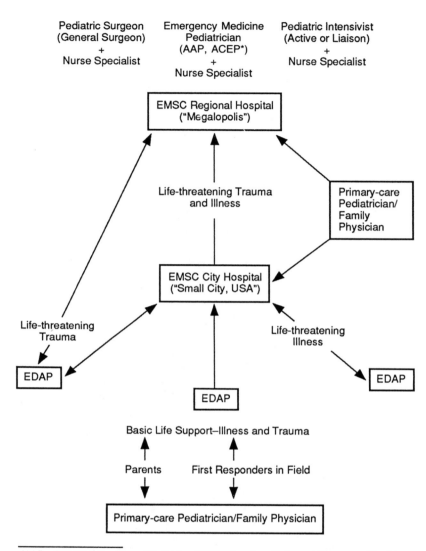

Pediatric Surgeon   Emergency Medicine   Pediatric Intensivist
(General Surgeon)   Pediatrician   (Active or Liaison)
       +   (AAP, ACEP*)   +
Nurse Specialist   +   Nurse Specialist
                           Nurse Specialist

EMSC Regional Hospital
("Megalopolis")

Life-threatening Trauma
and Illness

Primary-care
Pediatrician/
Family
Physician

EMSC City Hospital
("Small City, USA")

Life-threatening
Trauma

Life-threatening
Illness

EDAP   EDAP   EDAP

Basic Life Support–Illness and Trauma

Parents   First Responders in Field

Primary-care Pediatrician/Family Physician

*AAP = American Academy of Pediatrics; ACEP = American College of Emergency Physicians

Figure 1-1. The EMSC is an integrated system for the provision of care.

References

1. Harris, BH: Creating pediatric trauma systems. J Pediatr Surg 24:149–152, 1989
2. Tepas JJ, Ramenofsky ML, Barlow B et al: National Pediatric Trauma Registry. J Pediatr Surg 24:156–158, 1989
3. Haller, JA, Beaver B: A model: Systems management of life threatening injuries in children for the state of Maryland, USA. Intensive Care Med 15:S53–S56, 1989
4. Marganitt B, MacKenzie EJ, Haller JA Jr et al: Compliance with statewide regionalized pediatric trauma care system—trends over 8 years. Abstract submitted to the American Association for the Surgery of Trauma, 1989
5. Emergency medical services for children. In Haller JA (ed): Report of the 97th Ross Conference on Pediatric Research. Ross Laboratories, Columbus, Ohio, 1989
6. Seidel JS: EMS-C in urban and rural areas: The California experience. In Haller JA (ed): Report of the 97th Ross Conference on Pediatric Research. Ross Laboratories, Columbus OH, 1989

CHAPTER 2

The Economics of Pediatric Trauma Care

George D. Zuidema and Peter I. Buerhaus

A ccording to economic theory, the price of a commodity or service and the amount that is sold are determined by the factors affecting its demand and the factors affecting its supply. We do not intend to argue in this chapter that economic theory and its underlying assumptions can or should be applied to an analysis of the price and quantity of pediatric trauma care services that are "consumed." An economic framework is used because it provides a way to organize and discuss issues that affect the delivery of pediatric trauma care and that might not otherwise be described in this book. Furthermore, regardless of one's feelings about the desirability of adapting the principles of economics to the delivery of health care services, the infusion of economic behavior and market competition have become the hallmark of the 1980s, and there is little reason to suggest that this will not continue in the 1990s. It is important, therefore, that physicians and others concerned with developing the nation's pediatric trauma care system become aware of some of the economic forces likely to influence the quantity and quality of pediatric trauma care in the years ahead.

Demand for Pediatric Trauma Care Services

Examining the frequency of injuries provides a number of indicators of the total demand for pediatric trauma care services. The Congressional Office of Technology Assessment (OTA) estimated that each year 353,000 children are hospitalized nationally for traumatic injuries.[22] According to this estimate, each year about 1 in every 130 children is hospitalized because of injury. Expressed differently, before age 15, it can be expected that 1 child in every 9 will be hospitalized for a trauma-related injury. With respect to the number of emergency room visits owing to injuries, the OTA reports that children under age 15 make nearly 10 million emergency room visits each year. Of the total number of emergency room visits, Brill reports that 20 percent to 35 percent are made by children or adolescents; and during weekends and nights, children may comprise up to 40 percent of all emer-

Table 2-1. Percentage of Deaths from Injury and Other Causes

Cause	Age		
	1–4 yr	*5–14 yr*	*15–24 yr*
Injuries	46	55	79
Congenital anomalies	13	5	—
Cancer	7	14	5
Pneumonia/Influenza	3	—	—
Heart and liver disease	4	3	3
Other	27	23	13

(National Research Council and the Institute of Medicine: Injury in America: A continuing public health problem, p. 4. Washington, DC, National Academy Press, 1985)

gency room visits.[3] Moreover, Brill estimates that as many as 18 million children receive emergency room care and that 4 million (i.e., 22%) of these take place in rural hospitals with fewer than 100 beds.

Mortality rates for children are another indicator of the demand for pediatric trauma care. Table 2-1 shows that, between age 1 and 4 years, injuries account for nearly half (46%) of all deaths, more than half (55%) of the deaths in children age 5 to 14 years, and nearly four fifths (79%) of the deaths of children aged 15 to 24 years. Injuries account for far more deaths among children than do congenital anomalies, cancer, pneumonia and influenza, and heart disease.[12]

Table 2-2 lists the types of vehicle related and non-vehicle related accidents responsible for child mortality during 1984. Of the total number of fatalities, motor vehicle accidents caused the greatest number of deaths, particularly for ages 5 to 14 years. In addition, more children who were pedestrians were killed than were those who were occupants of a vehicle. With respect to the number of non-vehicle

Table 2-2 Number of Accidental Vehicle Deaths in Children, 1984

Type of Accident	Number of Fatalities by Age			
	< 1 yr	*1–4 yr*	*5–14 yr*	*Total*
Motor vehicle	161	977	1138	3401
Person killed:				
Occupant	115	349	420	1173
Pedestrian	14	502	321	1325
Pedal cycle	0	17	218	334
Motorcycle	0	4	98	124
Other	32	105	190	435
Air, rail and water craft	1	31	75	138
Other vehicle	0	9	24	50

(U.S. Congress, Office of Technology Assessment: Healthy children: Investing in the future, OTA-H-345. Washington, DC, U.S. Government Printing Office, 1988)

related fatalities, Table 2-3 shows that fires and burns were the leading cause of death, while other causes clustered into specific age groups: deaths from choking were most common in infancy; deaths from poisoning, falls, and drownings were more common in preschoolers; and deaths from firearms were rare in young children under age 5, but were the third leading cause of death in older children.

An economic approach to health care analysis also attempts to identify sociodemographic and economic characteristics of the population that affect the demand for pediatric trauma care. For example, when comparing accidental death rates by gender, the rate for boys is higher than that for girls.[2] A study on teenage mothers found that infants with very young mothers had significantly higher accident rates than infants with older mothers.[19] With respect to economic influences, persons with low incomes have higher injury-related mortality rates than wealthier persons,[16] which could indicate a lack of either general or health care-focused education or the resources to modify home or neighborhood environments.[22] And it has been shown that while there are more fire-related injuries among low-income urban-dwelling children, among low-income rural children more injuries are caused by farm equipment, poor roads, cars traveling at high speeds, and a lack of quick emergency response and transportation.[12, 16]

Injury prevention strategies are a final but important factor affecting the demand for pediatric trauma care. Three types of strategies to prevent injuries have been identified:[12,17] persuasion through educational programs (e.g., teaching the value of using seatbelts); regulating an individual's behavior (e.g., requiring use of infant car seats or the installation of smoke detectors); and automatic protection devices that help prevent injury through product or environmental design (e.g., equipping automobiles with passive restraints that automatically "seat belt" the occupant, or providing air bag restraints).

In general, education strategies designed to to prevent accidents are the least costly. Typically, they are implemented at the local level and have been shown to

Table 2-3. Non-Vehicle Accidental Deaths of Children, 1984

Type of Accident	Age			
	< 1 yr	1–4 yr	5–14 yr	Total
Fires and burns	139	641	508	1288
Drowning	70	556	494	1120
Choking	153	118	45	316
Firearms	0	39	259	298
Falls	28	86	68	182
Poisoning	21	77	56	154
Other	265	280	358	903

(U.S. Congress, Office of Technology Assessment: Healthy children: Investing in the future, OTA-H-345. Washington, DC, U.S. Government Printing Office, 1988)

have mixed effectiveness in reducing the number of accidental injuries and their severity.[22]

The second type of accident prevention strategy, regulating an individual's behavior, tends to be more effective than educational strategies, but generally involves higher costs. These costs are associated with educating the public about the behavior to be regulated, monitoring the behavior, and enforcing the regulated behavior through the imposition and collection of fines, or other penalties.[22] In addition, politicians bear another kind of cost—the risk of losing political support if the regulation involves loss of individual rights to a large number of voting constituents.[8] Despite these costs, regulatory strategies can decrease significantly the demand for pediatric trauma care. According to the OTA, between 1980 and 1984, state laws requiring use of infant car seats contributed to a 36 percent decrease in motor vehicle occupant deaths among children less than age 5 years.

The third prevention strategy, automatic protection, is frequently implemented by federal agencies. Often the cost of these programs is borne by manufacturers, but sometimes is paid for by the public. In some cases, the costs may not be high, especially when a firm considers the risk of losing a major market share if the public perceives the firm as objecting to a certain type of automatic protection device (e.g., opposing the federal law requiring child-proof caps for prescription medications). In other cases, the cost to the manufacturer is significant, as in the installation of air bags in automobiles. Depending on the nature of the product and market conditions, however, the manufacturer may be able to pass on part or all of the costs of automatic protection devices to the consumer.

While it is difficult to determine the number of accidental injuries prevented by these protection devices, there is evidence that deaths among children under age 15 have declined in recent years. For example, in 1975 there were 11,736 accidental deaths, but in 1984, almost 10 years later the number had dropped to 7,850 deaths.[22]

Supply of Pediatric Trauma Care

Using an economic framework to examine the supply of pediatric trauma care requires an analysis of the economic factors that affect the efficiency with which the supply side of the market is operating. The criteria used to judge the efficiency of the supply of pediatric trauma care services would address several questions. Is the total number of pediatric trauma centers optimal? Are the centers the right size and are they distributed geographically for ready access by a portion of the population that has been determined by professionals or selected to meet pertinent criteria? Are the centers producing their services at lowest possible cost? Do artificial barriers exist that prevent new pediatric trauma care centers from being developed? Unfortunately, it is impossible to discuss many of these issues in great detail in this chapter, though some of the more important ones are addressed later when the political-economic environment of health care is described. Supply issues are discussed in Chapter 3.

Costs of Pediatric Trauma Care and Federal Research Expenditures

Extrapolating from the results of a 1986 study involving Massachusetts children under age 19, the OTA estimated that the acute care costs of pediatric trauma for children in this age group were between $2 billion and $3.2 billion each year (1982 dollars). However, this figure does not include physician and non-hospital acute medical care costs. Parsons and associates estimated that in 1980 injury and poisonings accounted for a little more than 13 percent of all the acute medical care costs for children under age 17, or nearly $2 billion.[14] Neither estimate includes the costs of long-term pediatric care resulting from injuries. In light of the American Hospital Association (AHA) estimate that 100,000 children become permanently crippled each year, long-term care would drive the costs of pediatric trauma care considerably higher than the figures reported above.

A study by Munoz,[11] based on the outcomes of an economic model developed to estimate the total costs associated with pediatric trauma, provides the most detailed assessment of long-term costs of pediatric trauma. As shown in Table 2-4, the direct costs of *fatalities* refer to treatment-related costs, including emergency room services, in-patient care, physician and surgical services, administrative costs, and so forth. The direct costs of *nonfatal* accidents were those associated with rehabilitation services, care provided by attendants, structural alterations required in the homes of trauma victims, medical equipment, drugs, and the costs of rehospitalizations. Indirect cost estimates refer to earnings lost as a result of fatalities and nonfatal accidents. As Table 2-4 shows, boys account for twice as much in trauma care costs as girls, and the estimated total costs of pediatric trauma exceed the OTA's estimates by nearly 30 percent (i.e., $4.13 billion, compared to $3 billion).

In view of the magnitude of pediatric trauma costs, it is difficult to understand the relatively small amount of federal expenditures on injury-related research. For example, the National Institute of Health (NIH) spent $34.4 million on injury-related research in 1983, which was less than 2% of the NIH research budget.[12] Figure 2-1 shows total federal expenditures for nonmilitary research on injuries in 1983. Although the data are several years old and the actual dollar amounts have

Table 2-4. Total Costs of Pediatric Trauma Indexed to 1982 Dollars (In Millions)

Sex/Age	Fatalities		Nonfatalities		Total
	Direct	Indirect	Direct	Indirect	
Males: <14 yr	$17	$1487	$964	$291	$2759
Females: <14 yr	11	789	508	58	1366
					4125

(Munoz E: Economic costs of trauma: United States, 1982. J Trauma 24:237, 1984)

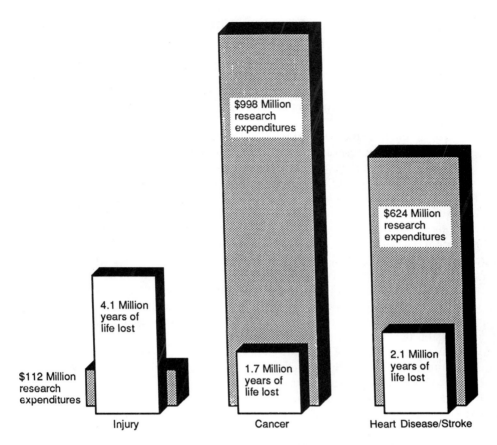

$998 Million research expenditures

$624 Million research expenditures

4.1 Million years of life lost

$112 Million research expenditures

1.7 Million years of life lost

2.1 Million years of life lost

Injury

Cancer

Heart Disease/Stroke

Figure 2-1. Years of life lost annually and federal research dollars for major causes of death (Injury in America: A continuing public health problem, p. 14. Washington, DC, National Academy Press, 1985)

changed, the relative proportions between years of life lost and dollars expended on research related to injury, cancer, and heart disease and stroke have remained unchanged. Given that the population of the United States is aging rapidly, and that retired individuals are dependent in large degree on the economic ability of younger generations to contribute financially to their well-being, increasing the amount of injury-related research and accident prevention programs could serve to increase the productivity of the younger generation.

The Political-Economic Environment of Pediatric Trauma Care

Pediatric trauma care is subject to the forces that shape and drive the larger, still developing, regional system of trauma care in the nation. The strength of pediatric trauma care and the entire trauma care system in the years ahead will depend in great part on how accurately future conditions are anticipated and on the development of strategies that successfully create opportunities and take effective advantage of unforeseen opportunities when they arise. With this perspective in mind, it is useful to examine some major forces that affect the nation's health care system and to identify their possible impact on the development of pediatric trauma care in the future.

During much of the 1980s, the federal government, and to a lesser extent state governments, were responsible for a great number of the initiatives that transformed the health care system. The major focus of federal initiatives has been the Medicare program, the federal program that administers and finances acute care hospital and physician care services provided to Americans who are 65 years and older. In 1989, Medicare will spend nearly $100 billion, which is equivalent to $274 million per day or almost $12 million per hour, on hospital and physicians costs for its beneficiaries. For most hospitals, 40 percent of revenues come from Medicare, a portion far exceeding that of any other individual payer. In its latest report to Congress, the Prospective Payment Assessment Commission notes that after several years of declining admission rates for persons over age 65, admissions for this group increased by nearly 2 percent in 1988. Over the next 3 decades, the number of persons over age 65 years, and especially those over age 85, is projected to grow faster than any other segment of the population.[15] This will mean a significant increase in the number of Medicare beneficiaries, who will consume more intensive acute care services. By the year 2000, it is estimated that Medicare will triple its spending to $320 billion per year.

Due to this projected growth, Medicare will continue to be the major focus of federal health care initiatives in the foreseeable future. As a result, the Medicare program will present irresistible opportunities to those responsible for constraining the federal budget. The President and Congress have 4 major areas for reducing the federal budget: entitlement programs account for roughly 48 percent of the budget (i.e., Social Security, Medicare, Medicaid); military spending takes 26 percent; interest on the federal debt requires 14 percent; and discretionary spending accounts for the remainder, or about 12 percent. Given the demands by health care and non–health-related interest groups for spending and the many worthwhile programs that deserve a portion of discretionary spending, it is obvious immediately that increasing the future amount of federal spending on trauma care will require a very challenging effort.

To reduce the budget, the President and Congress must take the money from some program. In the past, entitlement programs were spared as targets, but the 17 percent to 18 percent annual increase in Medicare spending of recent years has caused this to change. The most dramatic example of this shift in policymakers' attitudes was the implementation of the Medicare prospective payment system, now entering its seventh year, which pays hospitals according to diagnostic related groups (DRGs). The results of this prospective payment system have been impressive, as shown in Table 2-5. Compared to years of "double digit" increases, the rate

crease of economic competition within the health care industry. As in any competitively organized industry, health care firms must not only produce their services at the lowest cost so that they can be priced attractively, but must be equally sensitive to the quality of their services. If they are insensitive to both price and quality, then eventually they will go out of business because consumers will choose others who offer higher quality services at lower prices. Not surprisingly, a wide range of public and private organizations and philanthropic foundations have joined the health care industry in a vigorous quality-of-care research agenda, much of which is aimed at developing and evaluating methods for measuring, monitoring, and assuring the quality of health care. Not only is quality of care a major activity of formal organizations, but consumers are also interested in quality, expressed by demands to know the qualifications of health care providers and the type of care provided, be informed about the availability of alternatives, and receive assurance that someone is monitoring the quality of care they receive. Consumer interest in the quality of health care is likely to increase in the near term, especially as employers shift more health care costs to employees. Consequently, it can be anticipated that, like the rest of the health care system, the quality of care provided in pediatric trauma care centers will come under increasing scrutiny.

Still another development that may have spillover effects on pediatric trauma care centers is the reform in physician payments in which Congress and others have shown interest. As shown in Table 2-5, Medicare Part B spending for physicians has been rising rapidly for many years. In federal fiscal year 1990, Medicare spending on physician services will total nearly $38 billion. Because 75 percent of these dollars will come directly from the federal government's general revenues, it is not difficult to comprehend why Congress has targeted physician expenditures as a potential area for budget deficit reductions. While it is impossible to predict the effects on pediatric trauma care until the exact nature of physician payment reforms are known, it can be anticipated that growth in total outlays to physicians will decrease and there probably will be substantial redistribution of physician payments by specialty. These changes will certainly impose new pressures on pediatric trauma care, some of which are bound to affect negatively the availability of pediatric trauma surgeons and other physicians on the trauma care team.

In the future, Medicare increasingly will promulgate regulations that restrict payments to services judged to be medically effective, provided by the correct type of physician or other provider, and delivered in the correct health care setting at the lowest cost. Several studies are underway by the Health Care Financing Administration (which administers the Medicare and Medicaid programs) and other federal health agencies to identify the most cost-effective procedures provided by physicians. Presumably, this will lead to a limitation of the kind of procedures that will be paid for by Medicare and other payers who adopt its policies. Adding to these pressures will be the continuing expansion of peer review organizations and more stringent claims payments review by federal and private payers, especially Health Maintenance Organizations (HMOs). All of this means that the rationale underlying the expansion, quality, and cost effectiveness of pediatric trauma care centers, as well as the larger trauma care system, will be subjected to increasingly rigorous review.

Finally, two economic issues, which are already affecting the present supply of trauma care centers, will continue to exert pressure on the future supply of both adult and pediatric trauma care centers. First, as competition and cost containment pressures have intensified, health care providers' ability to "cross subsidize" services has gradually eroded. With price playing a more important role in their decisions, purchasers of health services (private and public) have become less willing to pay the artificially higher prices for health care that in the past gave providers the revenues to subsidize uncompensated care to the uninsured. Moyer reports that in 1987, fully 21.8 percent of children in the United States under the age of 15 did not have health insurance.[10] Because trauma care is expensive and often deals with gunshot and knife wounds (which are increasing in incidence among the pediatric population),[13] the financial losses for urban hospitals, already under great economic pressure, may become overwhelming. In Los Angeles County, for example, 10 trauma care centers have closed since 1985; in 1988, financial losses forced 2 trauma care centers to close in Chicago.[9] In both cities, substantial public funds have been required to keep the trauma care networks in operation.

The second economic pressure threatening access to trauma care is the closing of rural hospitals. Between 1980 and 1987, 201 of the nation's 2700 rural hospitals closed because of declining revenues resulting from fewer admissions, lower third party payments, higher levels of uncompensated care, and rising operating costs.[1] However, a recent report by the Department of Health and Human Services (HHS) Office of the Inspector General found that in only 8 of the 37 rural communities that experienced hospital closures in 1987 did residents have to travel more than 20 miles for emergency care.[6] While this suggests that rural hospital closure is not having a significant impact on access to trauma or emergency care, the picture may change if the prediction by the University of Illinois' Center for Health Services Research[1] that 600 more rural hospitals will close in the 1990s proves to be accurate.

References

1. American Hospital Association: Rural hospital closure: Management and community implications. Chicago, 1989
2. Baker SP, O'Neil B, Karpf RS: The injury fact book. Toronto, Heath and Company, 1984
3. Brill JE: Statement of American Academy of Pediatrics. Hearing before the Subcommittee on Health and the Environment of the Committee on Energy and Commerce, House of Representatives, September 18, 1987. Washington DC, U.S. Government Printing Office, 1988
4. Cales RH, Heilig R (eds): Trauma care systems: A guide to planning, implementation, operation and evaluation. Rockville, Maryland, Aspen Systems Corp., 1986

5. De Maria EJ, Merriam MA, Casanova LA et al: Do DRG payments adequately reimburse the costs of trauma care in geriatric patients? J Trauma 28:1244, 1988

6. Department of Health and Human Services, Office of the Inspector General: Hospital closure: 1987. OAI-04-89-00740. Washington DC, 1989

7. Eichelberger MR, Randolph JG: Progress in pediatric trauma. World J Surg 9:222, 1985

8. Feldstein PJ: The politics of health legislation: An economic perspective. Ann Arbor, Health Administration Press Perspectives, 1988

9. Glenn KJ: Trauma centers on a collision course. Med Health 43(insert), 1989

10. Moyer ME: A revised look at the number of uninsured Americans. Health Affairs 8:102, 1989

11. Munoz E: Economic costs of trauma, United States, 1982. J Trauma 24:237, 1984

12. National Research Council and the Institute of Medicine: Injury in America: A continuing public health problem. Washington DC, National Academy Press, 1985

13. Ordog GJ, Amitbah P, Wassenberger J, Balasubramaniam S: Pediatric gunshot wounds. J Trauma 27:1272, 1987

14. Parsons PE, Lichtenstein R, Berke SE: Costs of illness, United States, 1980: National medical care utilization and expenditure survey. National Center for Health Statistics, Public Health Services, Series C, Analytic Report No. 3, DHHS Publication Number 86-20403, Washington, U.S. Government Printing Office, 1986

15. Prospective Payment Assessment Commission: Medicare prospective payment and the American health care system: Report to the Congress. Washington DC, June 1989

16. Rivara FP: Epidemiology of childhood injuries. In: Preventing Childhood Injuries. Columbus, Ohio, Ross Laboratories, 1982

17. Robertson LS: Behavioral research and strategies in public health: A demur. Soc Sci Med 9:165, 1975

18. Schwab CW, Young G, Ciril I et al: DRG reimbursement for trauma: The demise of the trauma center (The use of ISS groupings as an early predictor of total hospital cost). J Trauma 28:939, 1988

19. Taylor B, Wadsworth J, Butler NR: Teenage mothering: Admission to hospital and accidents during the first 5 years. Arch Dis Child

20. Thomas F, Clemmer T, Larsen KJ, Menlove RL et al: The economic impact of DRG payment policies on air-evacuated trauma patients. J Trauma 28:446, 1988

21. Trunkey DO: Trauma. Sci Amer 249:28, 1983

22. U.S. Congress, Office of Technology Assessment: Healthy children: Investing in the future, OTA-H-345. Washington DC, U.S. Government Printing Office, 1988

23. Wise PH, Kotelchuck M, Wilson ML: Racial and socioeconomic disparities in childhood mortality in Boston. N Engl J Med 313:360, 1985

CHAPTER 3

Pediatric Trauma Hospital Organization

Max L. Ramenofsky

*I*njury in the pediatric age group continues to have a devastating effect in terms of mortality and long-term and permanent disabilities. Over the past decade, interest in the field of pediatric trauma has increased, as indicated by the development of pediatric trauma services within a variety of hospitals. This chapter describes organizational needs for hospitals interested in providing optimum care for the injured child.[1]

Generally, pediatric trauma care is provided in two types of hospitals: a children's hospital or an adult hospital that has a significant pediatric component. Not all children's hospitals are interested in or committed to providing pediatric trauma care. Similarly, not all hospitals that treat adult injuries will be able to meet the strict criteria for provision of state-of-the-art pediatric trauma care.

It is estimated that there are from 250 to 500 childhood injuries requiring hospitalization per one million population. This figure may be lower in population areas with a higher proportion of adults and may be higher in areas with a population with a younger mean age.

When developing a pediatric trauma hospital, two concepts must be borne in mind. First, the injured child must be transported rapidly to an appropriate definitive care center so that time is not lost in transport—time that could be used for the provision of care. Second, because the volume of significant injuries among children is only 25 percent of that for adults, the patient population of a hospital providing care must contain a significant number of injured children so that the evaluative and therapeutic skills of the pediatric trauma personnel are maintained and expanded. This has been referred to as the "critical mass" of injured children needed to maintain expertise.

The major document used by most hospitals wishing to obtain designation as a pediatric trauma hospital is the American College of Surgeons' *Resources for Optimal Care of the Injured Patient.*[1] The section of this document applying to the pediatric population is Appendix J.[1]

The organization of a pediatric trauma care hospital unit will be described in this chapter under the following topics: pre-planning, the trauma service, trauma resuscitation area, pediatric intensive care units, operating room, laboratory, rehabilitation, and quality assurance.

Pre-planning

In addition to devastating victims and their families, trauma can devastate a hospital that wishes to provide pediatric trauma care. Without agreement among hospital administration, medical staff, and nursing and ancillary personnel the effort is doomed to failure.

Trauma care is costly in terms of resources, personnel time, and space requirements. In order for a hospital to make an informed decision to provide pediatric trauma care, its administration must understand the degree of commitment required. Administrative understanding of the needs of a trauma program is one of the three key elements of pediatric trauma program development. The administration of a hospital must not waiver in its commitment to provide all of the resources necessary for a successful program. The second key element required is the commitment of the department of surgery. Surgeons are the core of the trauma service and must understand and agree to participate actively. Without this commitment no trauma service will succeed. Although trauma is a surgical disease, it is not treated solely by surgeons. A team approach to care of the injured child is necessary, and beneficial to the ultimate outcome—other surgical subspecialities and nonsurgical specialities must be involved. Thus, the commitment of pediatric orthopedics and neurosurgery, in addition to pediatric emergency medicine and pediatric critical care and anesthesia, are vital to the success of a pediatric trauma program. This need is invariable, whether the program is in a children's hospital or in an adult hospital with a significant pediatric component. The nursing service is the third key area of personnel. The nursing staff roles are discussed later in this chapter, but it must be mentioned here that nursing staff must have a similar wholehearted commitment to the trauma program.

Another important component that must be pre-planned and in place before a program starts providing pediatric trauma care is the method through which the program will communicate with both in-hospital and out-of-hospital care providers. This is an item of significant expense, but is mandatory for the successful functioning of a pediatric trauma program. It is vitally important that a pediatric trauma team be given as much advance notice as possible of the arrival of an injured child. This will not always be possible, but even when notice is extremely short, there must be a method by which the trauma team can be notified.

The methods for trauma communication vary among hospitals. Perhaps the most effective is a communication center staffed by communication specialists who use two-way voice communications with the trauma team and other nonclinical staff members. This two-way communication system allows for paramedic-to-trauma-surgeon and trauma-surgeon-to-paramedic communications. It also allows trauma surgeons to communicate with other members of the team when specific injuries are identified in the prehospital setting and thus to have appropriate specialists available upon arrival of the patient. Other methods of communication are trauma-team tone alerts and overhead voice paging.

The hospital area in which injured children will be treated must be pre-planned and functional prior to the start of a pediatric trauma care program. The trauma receiving/resuscitation room should be large enough to accommodate all trauma team members and portable or ceiling-fixed x-ray equipment. The room must also hold adequate equipment designed specifically for children.

Personnel working in the trauma resuscitation room and any part of the hospital where trauma patients are sent must be adequately trained to care for injured children. This includes, but is not limited to, training in the American College of Surgeons Advanced Trauma Life Support Course for Physicians (ATLS); trauma nurse courses, which are provided throughout the United States in a variety of settings; and critical care nursing courses. Many hospitals require that personnel who care for the injured participate satisfactorily in the Advanced Cardiac Life Support Course (ACLS) or the Pediatric Advanced Life Support Course (PALS) of the American Heart Association.

The pre-planning effort—and the program itself—is expensive to develop and implement. Frequently, administrators ask if the cost of setting up a pediatric trauma care program can be recouped. The answer is yes. By and large, pediatric trauma programs are different from most adult trauma programs in that there are a variety of third-party payment mechanisms commonly used by children's hospitals.

The final segment of the pre-planning phase that requires discussion here is designation of a hospital as a pediatric trauma center. Most areas of the United States that have trauma systems and pediatric trauma systems have gone through a formal process of development. This process begins with a state legislature or local municipality passing a trauma law. Most trauma laws mandate the development and designation of trauma centers. Once a trauma law is on the books, hospitals are asked if they wish to participate in the trauma system, and are required to meet a selected group of standards, such as those of the American College of Surgeons. Hospitals that wish to participate state in writing if they meet the standards. At this point, the lead agency within the state or municipality calls for a verification site visit. The verification site visit is made by members of the Verification Sub-Committee of the American College of Surgeons Committee on Trauma, which goes to each hospital and verifies whether or not it meets the standards. A report is generated by the sub-committee and sent to the designating authority. The authority, based on the findings of the Verification Sub-Committee, determines which hospitals will be designated as a trauma centers. Thus, designation is a political process and one that should not be undertaken solely by a hospital. When self-designation occurs, the overall care within a trauma system is generally handicapped.

The Trauma Service

Ideally, the trauma service is composed of numerous departments within a hospital, all working toward the common goal of providing optimum trauma care to the injured child. These services include the departments of surgery (pediatric surgery), pediatric orthopedics, pediatric neurosurgery, pediatric plastic surgery, pediatric urology, pediatric emergency medicine, pediatric anesthesia, pediatric critical care, the operating room, the laboratories, nursing services, social services, and rehabilitative medicine. All of these services affect the injured child at some point during the hospital stay. Thus, agreement on the roles to be undertaken by each area is vitally important to the functioning of the trauma service.

Generally, the pediatric trauma service is headed by a specific pediatric surgeon who is interested in the field of pediatric trauma. Administrative control may be housed within the department of pediatric surgery or within the hospital administration. Regardless of the specific arrangement, it is vital that the pediatric trauma service have an administrative component. This component is improved by the incorporation of a pediatric trauma coordinator, frequently a nurse interested in the field of pediatric trauma, who functions as the administrative liaison between the director of the pediatric trauma service, the administration, and nursing. It is through the director of the trauma service and the program coordinator that an organized system of quality assurance is maintained and updated constantly.

The injured child will generally be brought into the hospital system through the trauma resuscitation area, usually located in the emergency department. The choice of which trauma team members will meet the patient in the emergency room should be made according to the severity of injuries the child has sustained. Thus, the responding trauma team may vary from a complete team (including pediatric surgeon, pediatric emergency physician, pediatric critical care anesthesiologist, pediatric orthopedist and neurosurgeon, radiologist, laboratory technician, and social worker) to a scaled-down team, which may only consist of the pediatric surgeon and pediatric emergency physician.

The system of evaluating injury severity prior to the child's arrival at the hospital is key to the development of a smoothly functioning trauma resuscitation team. At the Benedum Pediatric Trauma Program of Children's Hospital of Pittsburgh, three levels of injury are identified. A level I trauma patient requires the full response of the pediatric trauma team, whereas the Level III injury requires the scaled-down pediatric surgeon and pediatric emergency physician team. Assignment of nursing personnel to the trauma team depends upon the severity of injury, identified before the child arrives.

Most pediatric trauma services admit injured children to one service for at least 24 hours, during which period all injuries are identified and initial therapeutic treatments initiated. When it becomes clear that a patient has a single-system injury, it is generally satisfactory to transfer the patient to a specific service. For example, a child who has been in a motor vehicle accident and has suffered a long bone fracture, but who cannot be said to be free from abdominal or central nervous system injury, should be admitted to the pediatric trauma service. After 24 hours, when it has become clear that only a single system has been injured (i.e., bone fracture), the patient can be transferred to the orthopedic service. In-hospital follow-up of this patient should be continued by the general pediatric trauma service, but the patient will become the primary responsibility of the orthopedic service.

It is clear that all children with multi-system injuries should be admitted to the general pediatric trauma service, where care can be directed by the director of the trauma service. When necessary operative procedures are outside the surgical expertise of the pediatric surgeon, the surgery can be arranged through agreements with the consulting services, (e.g., orthopedics, neurosurgery, plastic surgery, etc.) When a child has had multi-system injuries and all but one system has been resolved, the child can be transferred to the appropriate service.

Trauma Resuscitation Area and Procedures

In most hospitals, the emergency department is the area in which trauma resuscitation takes place. Regardless of this area's location, there are personnel, facilities, and equipment needs that must be met.

The personnel who staff the trauma resuscitation area generally will be a mix of physicians, nurses, and radiology and laboratory technicians. The area itself must be sufficiently large to accommodate the patient stretcher or bed; the pediatric trauma team, including physicians and nurses; and portable or ceiling-fixed x-ray equipment.

All physician personnel should be required to have participated in the ATLS course of the American College of Surgeons. As a general rule, the trauma team is headed by the most senior surgeon on the pediatric surgical call roster. Additional members of the trauma team include senior and junior surgical residents, pediatric emergency physicians, pediatric critical care physicians, and pediatric anesthesia physicians. Trauma resuscitation is directed entirely by the head of the pediatric trauma team, who is usually responsible for the initial assessment of an injured child.

Three mini-surgical teams are involved in a major pediatric trauma resuscitation. Airway control and maintenance is frequently handled by anesthesia or pediatric critical care physicians under the direction of the head of the trauma team. The pediatric emergency physician has specific evaluative and therapeutic duties assigned on the left side of the patient's torso, while the junior surgical resident is assigned duties on the patient's right side.

The secondary survey is carried out under the direction of the head of the trauma team and may be assigned to the surgical residents or the emergency physician. Each mini-surgical team has an assigned nurse to provide equipment and assistance. There is also a transcribing nurse in the resuscitation room, whose duty it is to keep an accurate spread-sheet record of all findings and of therapeutics provided.

When appropriate, a radiology technician obtains lateral cervical spine x-rays, chest x-rays, and pelvic films, as directed by the head of the trauma team. The tasks of blood drawing and starting intravenous lines are assigned to the mini-surgical teams by the head of the trauma team.

During the course of a trauma resuscitation and evaluation, the need for additional ancillary tests is identified by the head of the trauma team, who notifies the transcribing nurse of tests, such as a computed tomography (CT) scan, which will require the patient to be moved to another area.

The whole resuscitation and evaluation process is carried out within 20 minutes of the patient's arrival. Plans for transferring the patient to the next appropriate area for diagnosis or therapy are made within this timeframe. Agreements must be made with the departments of laboratory medicine and radiology for the availability of laboratory and radiologic technicians for the immediate evaluation of the injured child.

Pediatric Intensive Care Unit

In both a children's hospital and an adult hospital it is important that the pediatric intensive care unit be a separate and identifiable unit. It is not acceptable for there to be a mix of adult and pediatric patients in an intensive care unit.

The personnel in the pediatric intensive care unit will include the trauma surgeons, critical care medical specialists, other surgical and medical subspecialists, and nursing specialists. It is mandatory that the trauma surgeon and the trauma team provide continuity of care to the injured child recovering in the pediatric intensive care unit. Ancillary help is often valuable and generally can be obtained from the critical care service. Nursing personnel should be adequately trained in pediatric critical care nursing and should have successfully completed a critical care nursing course.

Equipment needed to appropriately monitor injured children includes a variety of electric monitors that have the capability to provide continuous readouts of arterial, venous, and intracranial pressure. In addition, end-expiratory CO_2 monitors and oxygen-saturation meters are required at the patient's bedside.

Operating Room

An operating room must be available immediately to a trauma patient, 24 hours a day, should the need arise. This mandates in-house operating room personnel, such as scrub nurses, circulating nurses, and operating room technicians. It is unacceptable for operating room teams to be on call from outside of the hospital.

Laboratory

The clinical laboratory for the injured child must have available all blood and fluid, chemical and electrolyte determinations. It is imperative that the laboratories be equipped to perform a variety of tests using a micro-volume method of blood collection. Laboratory facilities and services, including blood typing and cross matching, must be available 24 hours a day.

Rehabilitation

The rehabilitation or physical medicine service has a key effect upon the injured child. It is not sufficient for physical medicine to be an occasionally consulted service; it should be an intrinsic part of the trauma service and each day should evaluate the needs of any injured children who were admitted the previous day. A physiatrist or other appropriately trained individual is a vital part of the pediatric trauma service.

Quality Assurance

Assuring the quality of care provided to the trauma patient is a continuous process that requires a great deal of time and effort. Intrinsic to the concept of quality assurance is a trauma registry recording appropriate data on every trauma patient admitted to the hospital.[2] In a properly designed trauma registry, a variety of pre-programmed audit filters should be incorporated. Such audit filters include such items as unexpected return to the operating room, re-admission to hospital within 72 hours of discharge, unexpected death or survival based on a variety of scoring mechanisms, wound infections, prolonged stays in the intensive care unit, other surgical or nonsurgical complications, various pre-hospital errors of omission or commission, etc. By routinely reviewing all audit filters identified through the trauma registry and discussing their significance at a peer review conference, the quality of the system can be upgraded continually.

Part of the quality assurance process is a trauma conference, a true multi-disciplinary conference involving all surgical and medical specialties contributing to the care of injured children. This conference should be an educational and fact-finding conference in which errors are openly discussed and solutions sought and identified, and corrective action implemented. The conference should never be construed as a "witch hunt" or a "kangaroo court." In many, if not most states, a multi-disciplinary peer review trauma conference falls under the peer review right to privacy laws of the state and is considered not subject to subpoena.

Summary

A hospital desiring to provide pediatric trauma care must have the commitment of its administration and entire medical staff. Agreements with all involved departments and divisions within the hospital must be in place prior to the start of a pediatric trauma program. The administration of the hospital must understand and be firmly committed to the development of a trauma program. Without commitment and hospital-wide agreement on the necessity to provide trauma care, a trauma hospital and trauma service cannot function.

References

1. American College of Surgeons: Resources for Optimal Care of the Injured Patient. Chicago, October, 1989
2. Tepas JJ, Ramenofsky ML, Barlow B et al: National Pediatric Trauma Registry. J Ped Surg 24 (Feb):156–158, 1989

CHAPTER 4

Mediators of the Metabolic Responses to Trauma

Douglas W. Wilmore

S evere injury is characterized by a set of rather stereotypic responses. With restoration of circulatory volume, catabolic alterations occur. Net proteolysis is
accelerated, and this is manifest by the increased excretion of urinary nitrogen,
resulting in the rapid loss of body protein. Oxygen consumption rises and body
fuel oxidation shifts toward the use of body fat. Blood glucose is increased as hepatic gluconeogenesis is accelerated, providing essential fuel for reparative and
inflammatory tissues to optimize host defenses and ensure wound repair.

These post-injury responses are associated in time with alterations in the secretion of a variety of hormones and the elaboration of various cytokines, products of
the host's own cells. Studies in our laboratory over the past several years have
involved the infusion or stimulation of the mediators in normal volunteers in order
to assess the relative influence of individual factors on the post-traumatic response.

To investigate the role of hormones as mediators of the metabolic response
to injury, nine healthy male volunteers received a continuous 74-hour infusion of
the three "stress" hormones: cortisol, glucagon, and epinephrine.[1] As a control,
each subject received a saline infusion during another 4-day period. Diets were
constant and matched on both occasions. Hormonal infusion achieved plasma concentrations similar to those that have been observed following mild to moderate
injury. With this alteration in the endocrine environment, significant hypermetabolism, negative nitrogen and potassium balances, glucose intolerance, hyperinsu-
linemia, insulin resistance, sodium retention, and leukocytosis were observed.
Single hormone infusions indicated that these responses resulted from both
additive and synergistic interaction of the hormones. Triple hormone infusion
simulated many of the metabolic responses observed following mild to moderate
injury and other catabolic illness.

To evaluate the role of inflammatory mediators, we administered the sterile
inflammatory agent etiocholanolone, given daily by intramuscular injection for
three days. The effects of this agent were studied alone[2] and during the simultaneous infusion of the hormonal mixture.[3] Etiocholanolone injection alone resulted

in inflammation, fever, leukocytosis, increased serum C-reactive protein concentration, hypoferremia, and increased plasma activity of interleukin-1. Plasma concentrations of the counterregulatory hormones were normal and catabolic responses were not observed. When etiocholanolone was administered with hormonal infusion, there was a major interaction between the two stimuli: both mediators were necessary for the complete manifestation of the host response to injury.

To evaluate the effect of endotoxin on mediating these responses, seven normal volunteers received *E. coli* endotoxin (4 ng/kg) by intravenous infusion.[4] Saline was given during the control arm of the study. Endotoxin administration produced a response similar to an acute febrile illness, with flu-like symptoms, fever, tachycardia, hypermetabolism, and stimulation of stress hormone release. These events occurred shortly after the cytokine tumor necrosis factor (TNF) was detected in significant concentrations in the plasma.[5] Significant plasma elevations in interleukin-1 and gamma-interferon were not observed. Similar acute-phase and catabolic events could be reproduced in stable cancer patients receiving the intravenous infusion of TNF.[6]

Subsequent studies in animals have demonstrated that chronic sublethal infusion of TNF results in negative nitrogen balance, muscle atrophy, hepatic hypertrophy, and gastrointestinal hypoplasia. The effects of TNF on skeletal muscle appear to be mediated by the increased elaboration of glucocorticoids, for the pituitary–adrenal axis is stimulated by this cytokine, and muscle atrophy is not observed in adrenalectomized animals receiving TNF.[7] However, the effects of TNF on visceral organs are not mediated by increased corticosteroid elaboration, and these events may be the result of the direct effects of this cytokine or the induction of other cytokines, such as interleukin-6.

Thus, it appears that cytokines can stimulate the hormonal response to injury and mediate many of the acute-phase responses that occur following tissue damage and inflammation. Endotoxin can initiate or facilitate the generation of these substances, but antigenic responses or the stimulation of the complement cascade may also induce these changes. The use of antibodies to block the effects of endotoxin or the cytokine signals may be important approaches to modify the catabolic responses to injury.

References

1. Bessey PQ, Watters JM, Aoki TT, Wilmore DW: Combined hormonal infusions simulate the metabolic response to injury. Ann Surg 200:264–280, 1984
2. Watters JM, Bessey PQ, Dinarello CA et al: The induction of interleukin-1 in humans and its metabolic effects. Surgery 98:298–306, 1985
3. Watters JM, Bessey PQ, Dinarello CA et al: Both inflammatory and endocrine mediators stimulate host responses to sepsis. Arch Surg 121:179–190, 1986
4. Revhaug A, Michie HR, Manson JM et al: Inhibition of cyclooxygenase attenuates the metabolic response to endotoxin in humans. Arch Surg 123:162–170, 1988

5. Michie HR, Manogue KR, Spriggs DR et al: Detection of circulating tumor necrosis factor during endotoxemia in humans. N Engl J Med 318:1481–1486, 1988
6. Michie HR, Spriggs DR, Manogue KR et al: Tumor necrosis factor induces similar metabolic responses in humans. Surgery 104:280–286, 1988
7. Mealy K, van Lanschot J, Wilmore DW: Glucocorticoids mediate the catabolic effects of tumour necrosis factor during critical illness. Br J Surg 76:643, 1989

CHAPTER 5

Shock in Pediatric Trauma

Arnold G. Coran and John R. Wesley

S hock in infants is similar to shock in adults, but also has many important differences in both presentation and treatment. This chapter focuses on how and why shock is different in infants and children and reviews the application of modern concepts in shock management to the specific requirements of the pediatric trauma victim.

Infants present a number of unique risk factors for shock that are not seen in adults. These include problems related to the process of birth, certain hematologic abnormalities, congenital anatomic defects, nutritional deficiencies, immunological immaturity, and temperature instability. Because of their small size, infants and children are less tolerant of therapeutic errors than adults. However, there are certain risk factors common among adults that are rare in children, such as coronary artery disease, myocardial infarction, and pulmonary embolism.[1] Because pediatric patients have not been exposed to the ravages of time and self-destructive life styles, they generally respond more quickly to antishock measures and with optimal treatment have a much better prognosis.

As with adults, proper shock management in the pediatric age group cannot be delivered without an appreciation of the underlying cause. However, shock does seem to be a common final pathway to the preterminal stage of many dissimilar diseases and as such requires rapid therapeutic intervention, frequently given without a firm diagnosis. The common denominator in most forms of shock is a failure of cellular function, usually on the basis of inadequate perfusion of vital tissues, depriving them of oxygen and other nutrients.

Classification

A classification of shock based upon etiology is presented in Table 5-1, and is similar to that used by a number of clinical investigators.[1,2,3] This classification serves well for infants and children, although specific causes under each broad classification are frequently different from those commonly seen in adults. The importance of a good history and physical examination cannot be overemphasized, and together with certain laboratory tests form the basis for classification and subsequent therapy.

Table 5-1. Etiologic Classification of Shock

Hypovolemia
Cardiac failure
Bacteremia
Hypersensitivity
Neurogenic causes
Vascular obstructing lesion

Hypovolemic shock is the most common form of shock in the pediatric age group and is most often the result of dehydration and desalting fluid loss through diarrhea or vomiting. It is also the most common form of shock in the pediatric trauma victim and is usually caused by hemorrhage. In newborn infants, however, septic shock is probably more common than hypovolemic shock. Shock can also occur as the result of massive fluid extravasation from large burns, peritonitis, or severe trauma. Unique causes of hemorrhagic shock in the newborn include avulsion of the umbilical cord,[4] occult hemorrhage secondary to coagulation deficiencies and birth trauma,[5] transplacental hemorrhage from fetus to mother,[6] and twin-to-twin transfusion syndrome.[7]

Cardiogenic shock is uncommon in pediatric patients, but may occur in children with acute arrhythmias or congestive heart failure, or in surgical patients after open heart surgery. It occurs infrequently following blunt trauma to the chest in children. The underlying defect is poor myocardial function despite adequate venous return, resulting in diminished cardiac output.

Sepsis is common in newborn infants, particularly premature and small-for-gestational-age infants, and shock should be suspected whenever sepsis is present. It is also fairly common in older children who have suffered from blunt and penetrating trauma to the abdomen, especially if bowel perforation has occurred. Bacteremic shock is caused by toxins released into the bloodstream by microbial agents, most commonly endotoxins shed by gram-negative bacteria. Although the mechanism is not completely understood, it is known that endotoxin has a direct effect on the heart and blood vessels, increases vascular permeability, activates the coagulation system, severely deranges intermediary metabolism, and releases endogenous vasoactive substances, including kinins,[8] endorphins,[9] and prostaglandins.[10]

Hypersensitivity shock is an extreme form of allergy leading to sudden vascular collapse and is often associated with asthma-like symptoms and severe bronchial constriction. It may be seen after injection of a drug or, less commonly, after an insect bite. The mechanism is a direct toxin effect plus loss of intravascular volume through tissue edema, leading to a hypovolemic type of shock.[1,5]

Neurogenic shock is the result of severe impairment of the central nervous system (CNS) caused by trauma or by the administration of certain CNS-blocking or depressant drugs. The mechanism is a loss of vasomotor tone leading to circulatory failure because of a disproportion between vascular volume and vascular capacity. The intravascular volume is normal, but the capacity of the vascular system is greatly expanded, especially on the venous side. This leads to a rapid fall in intravenous pressure and a diminished cardiac output. Remarkable improvement follows expansion of vascular volume.[1,5]

Vascular obstruction leading to shock is rare in pediatric patients, and includes pulmonary emboli;[11] spontaneous or traumatic thrombosis of the inferior vena cava, renal veins, or distal aorta; and disseminated microvascular obstruction associated with consumption coagulopathy.[5] The common denominator is a major impediment to venous return, resulting in decreased cardiac output.

Phases of Shock

Although diverse in its causes, shock is progressive with common characteristics that lead to a useful division into three clinical phases: compensated, uncompensated, and irreversible. In phase 1, an insult has occurred, but compensatory mechanisms maintain an adequate blood pressure, although ominous shifts in tissue perfusion are apparent. The classic clinical manifestations of this stage include pallor, clammy skin with cool extremities, apprehension, and tachycardia; all are a result of increased sympathetic activity. If the insult continues, or if compensatory mechanisms fail, then phase 2 ensues. In the second or uncompensated phase, blood is diverted to vital organs at the expense of reduced perfusion elsewhere, leading to regional ischemia, anaerobic metabolism, acidosis, and cellular injury. The patient becomes progressively obtunded as the circulation fails, poor skin turgor and dry mucous membranes signal fluid loss, and oliguria reflects diminished renal perfusion. Jaundice, petechiae, and peripheral or local edema may be part of the general appearance. Although major organs may be damaged at this phase, the deteriorating clinical situation is still amenable to corrective therapy. If this phase is left untreated, there is continued decompensation to phase 3, the final phase of shock—irreversible tissue damage and death despite therapy that may temporarily return cardiovascular measurements to normal levels. "The skilled clinician recognizes Phase 1, reverses Phase 2, and prevents Phase 3."[1]

Clinical Manifestations

In evaluating an infant or child in shock, the examiner must first be aware of the normal vital signs and urinary output in these age groups. Not knowing that they differ from adult norms may lead to an incorrect diagnosis of shock (Tables 5-2 and 5-3). The classical clinical manifestations of a patient in shock have already been alluded to in discussion of the phases of shock. Several special considerations are important for effective diagnosis and treatment of infants and children.

First, the infant with inadequate tissue perfusion may exhibit a unique syndrome called "sclerema neonatorum"—a diffuse, rapidly spreading, nonedematous, tallow-like hardening of subcutaneous tissue during the first few weeks of life.[12] Until the mid-1960s, sclerema was looked upon as a rare disease of unknown

Table 5-2. Normal Vital Signs in Infants and Children

	Pulse (per min)	Blood pressure (mm Hg)	Respiratory rate (per min)
Infant	160	80	40
Toddler	140	90	30
Adolescent	120	100	20

cause with an almost uniformly fatal prognosis. Because of isolated reports of therapeutic success with steroids, antibiotics, and transfusions, steroid therapy was regarded as possibly specific for this unusual disorder. It now appears more likely that sclerema represents a state of poor perfusion in shock that may have a number of underlying causes.[3] The infant's subcutaneous tissues undergo a unique pathological change, but otherwise the basic pathophysiology appears similar to shock syndromes in older patients.

Second, the pulse rate of a patient in shock is generally thought of as being elevated. This is usually, though not always, true, and perhaps has been overemphasized in adults as well as in children. Weil and Shubin analyzed the heart rate of 25 patients with shock caused by myocardial infarction and found that the average rate was essentially the same as the rate in 125 patients in whom myocardial infarction was not complicated by shock.[13] Evaluation of heart rate as an indicator of cardiovascular decompensation is even more complicated in infants, in whom the normal range is much more variable than in adults. Therefore, it is unreliable to use isolated determinations of an infant's heart rate as an index of impending circulatory collapse. Instances of sudden cardiovascular collapse have been reported without the warning of a noticeable elevation in heart rate, and bradycardia usually develops in newborn infants during the early phase of shock.[14]

Third, reduced blood pressure is also generally regarded as an important component of the shock syndrome, although it is possible to have serious forms of shock with elevated blood pressure and associated increased vascular resistance. The infant or small child in a state of shock is difficult to evaluate because it is technically difficult to measure blood pressure accurately under conditions of circulatory decompensation. Moreover, the range of normal blood pressure changes considerably over the first two weeks of life, and mean pressures that would be considered shock levels for an adult can be normal pressures for an infant. Moss

Table 5-3. Urinary Output in Infants and Children

	Ml/kg body wt/hr
Infant	2
Toddler	1–2
Adolescent	0.5

and associates reported normal values obtained by umbilical artery catherization that range from 44/24 mm Hg to 84/54 mm Hg in premature infants, and 53/33 mm Hg to 91/61 mm Hg in full-term infants.[15,16] This wide variability in normal values underscores the importance of following trends with serial pressure measurements because individual determinations may appear to be alarmingly low. The difficulties in clinical evaluation of such basic measurements as pulse and blood pressure emphasize the importance of precise methods of clinical monitoring.

Monitoring

Monitoring the pediatric patient in shock has the following four broad goals: find the etiologic factors and cardiorespiratory pattern helpful in diagnosis, prognosis, and treatment; permit continuous assessment of vital organ function; provide a means of assessing the response to therapy; and minimize the frequency of complications by detecting correctable problems early, thereby facilitating rapid resolution.

Measurements for monitoring shock in infants and children are listed in Table 5-4. In general, these are the same measurements that are monitored in adults, but the technical aspects of measurement are frequently more difficult and exacting in the pediatric age group.

Table 5-4. Monitoring Infants and Children in Shock

Essential measurements		Desireable measurements
Arterial pressure	Hematocrit	Pulmonary artery pressure
Central venous pressure	WBC	Pulmonary wedge pressure
Heart rate	Differential count	Cardiac output
Continuous EKG	Platelet count	Lactic acid
Respiratory rate	Clotting time	Urine osmolality
Rectal temperature	Fibrinogen	Liver function tests
Surface temperature	Partial thromboplastin	Bilirubin
	time	SGOT
Abdomen	Sodium	SGPT
Extremities	Potassium	LDH
Inspired O_2 concentration	Chloride	Amylase
Arterial pO_2	BUN	Transcutaneous O_2, CO_2
Arterial O_2 saturation	Creatinine	
Arterial pCO_2	Glucose	
Arterial pH	Urine sugar	
Base excess	Bacterial cultures	
Fluid input	Blood	
Urine output	Urine	
Serial roentgenograms—chest	Sputum or tracheal	
and disease-specific	aspirate	
Daily weight	Specific local infections	

Standard blood pressure techniques with a cuff are unreliable in vasoconstricted infants. Because of the large range of extremity size in the pediatric age group, cuffs are frequently either too large or too small relative to the circumference of the extremity, and mechanical errors frequently occur.[17] In addition, intravascular arterial pressure measured directly by strain-gauge transducers may be considerably higher than cuff pressure obtained by auscultation or palpation because of the initially higher vascular resistance in some patients with shock, which dampens or eliminates the Korotkoff sounds or radial pulses.[10] Failure to recognize that low cuff pressure does not necessarily indicate arterial hypotension may lead to dangerous errors in therapy. Therefore, for a sick, unstable child with a need for frequent or continuous blood pressure monitoring, we insert a radial or umbilical arterial line and measure the pulse and mean arterial pressure directly.[18] The line is also used for obtaining arterial blood gas tensions, pH, and other important blood chemistries with minimal discomfort to the patient. Transcutaneous O_2 monitoring is a new technique for assessing arterial oxygenation.

Although central venous pressure (CVP) is technically more difficult to obtain in the infant and child than it is in the adult, it has the same clinical usefulness and probably the same physiologic significance. As has been emphasized by many authors, changes in central venous pressure can be used as an index of the heart's ability to pump the volume of fluid presented to it, and changes in CVP are not an index of the circulating blood volume, the cardiac output, or the size of the venous reservoir.[5,19,20] The subclavian approach is the usual route we use for central venous access. In infants, subclavian cannulation is much more difficult and hazardous than in older children, and the external jugular vein or internal jugular vein is preferred for cannulation. It is rarely feasible to thread a catheter from the antecubital space up the basilic vein and into the superior vena cava in an infant, although a proximal saphenous vein cutdown can be used for access to the inferior vena cava. Subclavian catheterizations in an infant requires experience and careful attention to technical details if serious complications are to be avoided. A closed syringe-and-needle system must be used to avoid pneumothorax and air embolism. The insertion maneuver must not incorporate any change of needle direction once the skin has been penetrated, and to avoid tearing vessels the needle must be completely withdrawn before changing direction.

Although usually not required for management of shock, except in cardiogenic shock or cardiac dysfunction, a pulmonary artery catheter (pediatric Swan-Ganz) can be placed to measure pulmonary arterial pressure and pulmonary wedge pressure (PWP). Because many patients with cardiogenic shock or cardiac dysfunction show poor correlation between pressure on the right side of the heart (CVP) and pressure on the left side of the heart (PWP), both measurements are needed to manage successfully volume replacement and inotropic and chronotropic drug administration.[21] In addition, these catheters are available with an incorporated thermister, which can be used for measuring cardiac output by use of the principle of thermodilution. The thermodilution technique compares favorably with more traditional methods for estimating cardiac output. Determinations can be made frequently and rapidly by injecting a room-temperature physiologic saline solution as the indicator.[22] No blood need be withdrawn from the patient, and small volumes of indicator cause no significant blood temperature changes even in patients of less than 10 kg body weight. These catheters are inserted percutaneously using the Seldinger technique, with the femoral vein being the favored venous entry site. A portable fluroscopic image intensifier facilitates placement, although measuring the pulmonary artery pressure and noting the difference after the catheter balloon tip is inflated and "floated" into the pulmonary wedge position is generally sufficient.[21]

Continuous monitoring of heart rate with an oscilloscope to display rhythm patterns and a cardiotachometer for ease of recording is essential for all shock patients. Reliable miniaturized adhesive leads are available and convenient even for premature infants.

Temperature monitoring is extremely important in infants and small children. Protection against thermal stress is often overlooked in the urgency of performing a variety of procedures and therapeutic maneuvers for a patient in shock. In addition to underdeveloped thermoregulatory mechanisms, premature infants have a much higher ratio of body surface area to total body mass than older children or adults, resulting in greater heat loss. Negative thermal balance can increase oxygen consumption and energy expenditure several times over and prove highly detrimental, defeating other therapeutic attempts to counter shock in an infant.[23] In addition to core temperature, surface temperature monitoring is important in that peripheral surface temperature is related to the state of perfusion. An infant well perfused has a small temperature gradient between the central portions of his or her body and the periphery.[5]

As with adults, frequent measurement of urine volume in infants and children is a useful index of renal perfusion and function. Infants and children are less likely than adults to retain urine on the basis of immobility or mechanical problems, and they void much more frequently (up to 20 times a day for a newborn infant). The more delicate and short urethera in the infant and small child makes complications of uretheral instrumentation and induced infection more likely. For these reasons, urine should be collected by external appliances when feasible. If this is unsatisfactory, however, catheter drainage must be used so that urine output can guide appropriate therapy.

Laboratory measurements should always include serial hematocrit readings, white blood cell counts, and differentials. Trends in the hematocrit reading are useful if the examiner takes into account the time lag necessary for dilutional changes. Serum sodium, potassium, and chloride levels must be monitored for adequate fluid management. Blood urea nitrogen and serum creatinine levels are followed as part of the renal evaluation, and osmolarity of both serum and urine is desirable if available. Serial blood glucose determinations are particularly important in newborn infants in a state of shock because of the increased frequency of hypoglycemia and its complications. Arterial blood pH and gas partial pressure measurements are important to adjust respiratory settings and to provide measurements for correcting respiratory and metabolic acidosis. Blood lactate levels are also desirable as a measure of metabolic acidosis and as an index of the severity of shock.

Ongoing evaluation of the coagulation system is important because of the known changes in coagulability with certain types of shock, and because heparin anticoagulant therapy may be essential in shock associated with disseminated intravascular coagulation.[24] Newborn infants, however, are rarely heparinized because of their increased risk of intracranial bleeding under conditions of physiologic stress. Serial cultures of blood, urine, and any other focus of infection must be followed carefully to guide antibacterial therapy. Serial chest roentgenograms and other appropriate roentgenologic imaging relevant to the clinical problem area are always a part of shock management. Serial enzyme studies, including liver function tests, are a useful measurement of organ function and the severity of shock injury. In that infants and children have unique metabolic requirements because of their need for body growth and CNS development, we have started to measure resting energy expenditure by means of indirect calorimetry. This allows for provision of more appropriate calorie levels on a daily basis, and is particularly important during the patient's weaning from a respirator and during recovery from shock.[25]

Treatment

The usual approach of diagnosis first and treatment later may not be appropriate in shock. Rather, physicians must initiate orderly treatment immediately and gain insight into the cause of the patient's illness as the treatment proceeds. The child's own compensatory mechanism and defenses are generally inadequate to protect those organs with little margin for interruption of oxygen and nutrients. Cells deprived of oxygen and energy rapidly reach an irreversible state of injury, and cell death may proceed even if circulation is later restored. Therefore, a plan directed at the pathology common to all types of shock allows prompt treatment in this life-threatening condition. The plan includes first correcting hypoxia by appropriate airway management, stopping massive hemorrhage, gaining vascular access, splinting unstable fractures, administering fluids and appropriate drugs, identifying sepsis and starting antibiotics, considering early administration of steroids, and monitoring the patient as described in the previous section. Outlines for managing the most commonly encountered forms of shock, hypovolemic (including hemorrhagic) and septic, are provided in Figures 5-1 and 5-2.

Airway

The patient's airway and oxygen status should receive first and immediate attention. A low threshold should be maintained for early intubation. Early and frequent monitoring of arterial blood gases and *p*H is important. Abnormalities in oxygenation, ventilation, and acid–base balance can adversely affect cardiovascular perfor-

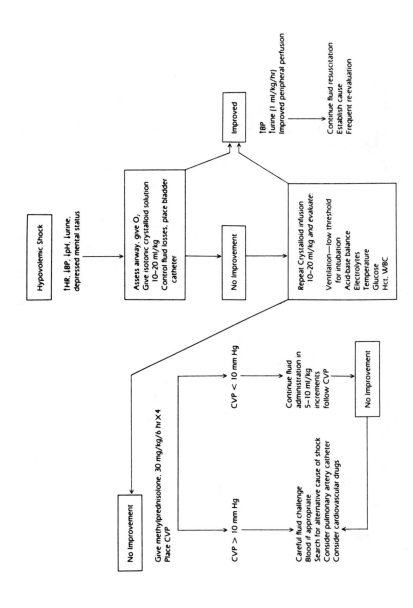

Figure 5-1. Algorithm for the treatment of hypovolemic and hemorrhagic shock.

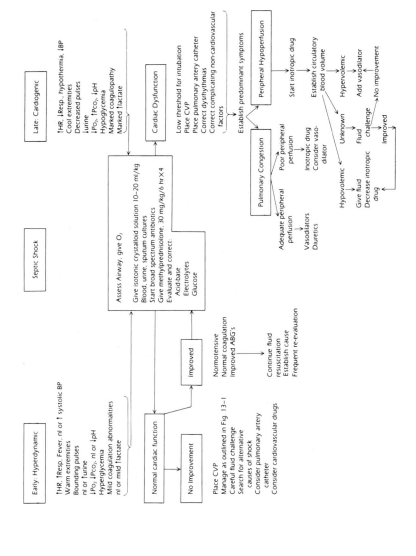

Early: Hyperdynamic

↑HR, ↑Resp. Fever, nl or ↑ systolic BP
Warm extremities
Bounding pulses
nl or ↑urine
↓Po₂, ↓Pco₂, nl or ↓pH
Hyperglycemia
Mild coagulation abnormalities
nl or mild ↑lactate

Septic Shock

Late: Cardiogenic

↑HR, ↓Resp. hypothermia, ↓BP
Cool extremities
Decreased pulses
↓urine
↓Po₂, ↑Pco₂, ↓pH
Hypoglycemia
Marked coagulopathy
Marked ↑lactate

Assess Airway, give O₂

Give isotonic crystalloid solution 10–20 ml/kg
Blood, urine, sputum cultures
Start broad spectrum antibiotics
Give methylprednisolone. 30 mg/kg/6 hr × 4
Evaluate and correct:
  Acid-base
  Electrolytes
  Glucose

Improved

Normotensive
Normal coagulation
Improved ABG's

Continue fluid resuscitation
Establish cause
Frequent re-evaluation

Normal cardiac function

No Improvement

Place CVP
Manage as outlined in Fig 13–1
Careful fluid challenge
Search for alternative
  causes of shock
Consider pulmonary artery
  catheter
Consider cardiovascular drugs

Cardiac Dysfunction

Low threshold for intubation
Place CVP
Place pulmonary artery catheter
Correct dysrhythmias
Correct complicating non-cardiovascular
  factors

Establish predominant symptoms

Pulmonary Congestion

Adequate peripheral perfusion

Vasodilators
Diuretics

Poor peripheral perfusion

Inotropic drug
Consider vaso-dilator

Hypovolemic

Give fluid
Decrease inotropic drug

Unknown

Fluid challenge

Improved

Peripheral Hypoperfusion

Start inotropic drug

Establish circulatory blood volume

Hypervolemic

Add vasodilator

No improvement

Figure 5-2. Algorithm for the treatment of septic shock.

38

mance and systemic oxygen transport, and should be corrected early and reassessed frequently.

The lung is one of the most sensitive organs in shock; respiratory failure can develop rapidly, and if support is delayed until respiratory failure is obvious, mortality is greatly increased.[26,27] The use of paralytic or sedative drugs will further reduce the oxygen cost of breathing and enhance positive pressure ventilation.[28]

Vascular Access

Simultaneously with airway management, adequate vascular access must be established. The traditional saphenous vein percutaneous insertion or cutdown in infants and small children is rapidly performed in experienced hands, and is reliable for administration of blood and crystalloid at rapid rates. However, a central venous line is also desirable for ready measurement of CVP, which is a helpful variable to follow during fluid resuscitation in a pediatric trauma victim. Serial CVP measurements together with pulmonary wedge pressures obtained from a balloon-tipped pulmonary artery catheter are necessary for successful treatment of patients in the later phases of shock. As has already been described, the variability and potential unreliability of cuff blood pressures make it advisable to maintain a low threshold for inserting a radial or umbilical arterial line to follow mean arterial pressure accurately, and to have ready access for arterial blood gas and *p*H measurements.

Fluid Administration

Once dependable venous access has been established, a fluid challenge of 10 ml/kg to 20 ml/kg is administered rapidly, and systemic arterial pressure response to the fluid challenge is assessed. If shock is on the basis of hemorrhage, a blood sample is sent immediately for typing and cross-matching, and blood is administered as soon as it is available. If systemic arterial pressure does not return to and remain at normal levels for the patient's age following the fluid challenge, additional volumes are infused and titrated against CVP as outlined in Figures 5-1 and 5-2. Initially CVP levels are followed because of the greater ease in obtaining these measurements. If circulatory instability persists after achieving adequate CVP levels (10–15 mm Hg), however, a balloon-tipped, flow-directed pulmonary artery catheter should be placed to obtain pulmonary wedge pressure, which more accurately reflects filling pressure of the left heart and allows measurement of cardiac efficiency by thermodilution cardiac output.

As has been demonstrated by several investigators, one of the most important therapeutic maneuvers in shock is to restore an adequate circulatory volume with a physiologic salt solution that has some oncotic pressure and yet is readily reabsorbed from the extravascular "third space" once the integrity of leaky capillary beds has been restored.[29,30] Lactated Ringer's solution or lactated Ringer's solution with 5 percent albumin has the best therapeutic record as the initial fluid choice both clinically and experimentally.[14,29,31,32] However, subsequent fluid resuscitation must take into account what type of fluid has been lost, the specific underlying physiologic problems, the need for maintaining an adequate oxygen-carrying capacity for the patient, and the physiologic actions of each fluid type.[30]

Fluid replacement programs should include an allowance for extracellular deficit as well as extra free water in the form of glucose solution to enhance renal tubular flow and urinary output. This usually starts out as a calculated fluid infusion of 110 percent to 125 percent of the estimated losses, but may require a threefold or greater increase before changes in CVP are observed. While a CVP of 10 mm Hg is generally regarded as a safe upper limit before inotropic cardiotonic drugs are initiated, it is most important to look for a change in CVP in response to the fluid infusion rather than look for an absolute value.

Corticosteroids

If septic shock has been diagnosed or is strongly suspected, then a large pharmacologic dose of short-acting steroids should be administered. Steroids act to stabilize cellular and subcellular (lysosomal) membranes, and block complement (C_{3a}, C_{5a}) as well as the synthesis of certain prostaglandins and endorphins recently found to be important mediators in shock.[9,33-35] An appropriate short-acting steroid dose is 30 mg/kg of methylprednisolone sodium succinate (Solumedrol).[36,37] This should be infused over 30 minutes and continued every 6 hours for no longer than 12 to 18 hours in order to avoid the deleterious tissue anti-inflammatory effects of steroids administered for longer periods. Broad-spectrum antibiotics, including an aminoglycoside, should be started at the same time. The same inflammatory systems responsible for defending against bacterial invasion into tissues can produce septic shock when activated intravascularly by bacterial endotoxins, and hence early steroid treatment is essential in order to be predictably effective.[38,39] However, a recent, large cooperative study of the use of high-dose methylprednisolone in the treatment of septic shock in adults has shown no benefit and no improved survival.[40,41] Nevertheless, we still recommend the use of high-dose corticosteroids under certain conditions. Because there is no reliable biochemical marker for early septic shock, clinical findings are important and include extremes of body temperature, altered mental status, unexplained edema, leukopenia, thrombocytopenia, and tachypnea or hypoxemia with development of a metabolic acidosis. In the neonate thrombocytopenia is often the first evidence of impending septic shock.[42]

Other Drugs

The clinical history and physical examination will usually lead the physician to administer cardiac drugs if myocardial failure is a major contributor to shock. If the CVP is elevated in the presence of inadequate peripheral perfusion, specific measures must be directed toward improving myocardial efficiency. Any of the following may be indicated, depending on the clinical situation: increased inspired oxygen, drugs to correct an abnormal rhythm or rate, digitalis preparations,[43] iso-proterenol,[1] dopamine,[44] or dolbutamine. The latter two drugs stimulate cardiac and peripheral beta receptors that have positive inotropic and selective vasodilator effects, depending on the dose, which must be carefully regulated.[45] Dopamine is particularly useful in low doses (less than 10 ug/kg/min) to dilate renal and mesenteric vascular beds and in conjunction with appropriate volume therapy is effective in helping to restore renal and gastrointestinal circulation.[45,46] As has been alluded to previously, bicarbonate infusion in appropriately calculated doses represents a temporary maneuver to acutely correct low pH so that myocardial contractility and systemic enzyme function can be optimized.[41] Bicarbonate rarely maintains arterial pH unless perfusion and oxygenation are simultaneously corrected.

Other promising drugs that have been shown to be effective for the treatment of shock in experimental or clinical situations are: naloxone (an endorphin antagonist),[47-50] antiserum to endotoxin,[51] indomethacin (a prostaglandin inhibitor), [52] ibuprofen (a prostaglandin inhibitor),[5,53-55] and prostacyclin.[56] The latter is a prostaglandin that, in contrast to a number of prostaglandins with deleterious inflammatory effects, exerts a number of beneficial effects in endotoxin shock in animals, including vasodilation, stabilization of lysosomal membranes, reduction of platelet aggregation, and suppression of thromboxane formation.[56] Many of these new and experimental drugs have not yet been tried in immature experimental animals or in pediatric patients. As more is learned about the pathophysiology of the several types of shock in the pediatric age group, drugs with increasingly more specificity can be administered to block, reduce, or reverse the shock syndrome.

New Directions

Continued progress in experimental shock research and clinical application in the pediatric age group will require increasingly more sophisticated monitoring devices and a means of identifying patients at risk for hypovolemic or septic shock at an earlier time, when they can be treated with a greater expectation of success. One of the new monitoring devices on the horizon for clinical application is the micro pH probe.[57] This probe allows constant read-out of tissue pH by a micro-probe inserted percutaneously—a good indicator of tissue perfusion.

More sophisticated use of drugs to alleviate the shock syndrome is already happening, and as the role of specific mediators, certain prostaglandins, endorphins, complement factors, endotoxins and oxygen radicals[58] become better understood, blocking agents will be developed to counteract their effects. For example, although no effective parenteral antiprostaglandin drugs are available for clinical use at present, they are being developed with the goal of maximizing the intravascular anti-inflammatory effect in the second phase of shock, especially septic shock, without impairing the host's tissue-based anti-inflammatory and immune mechanisms.[34] On the basis of experimental shock research, there is little question that large doses of short-acting steroids are effective in the first and early second phases of shock because they inhibit the synthesis and occupy the receptor sites of a number of deleterious prostaglandins, endorphins, and complement factors. The problem with the use of corticosteroids is that they are only effective early and briefly, and interfere with important host defenses, especially those against microbial invasion.[59]

When the usual medical means of treating shock in the newborn with severe respiratory distress have failed, we have placed the infant's lungs at complete rest by means of extracorporeal membrane oxygenation (ECMO), and have been encouraged by its success in carefully selected patients.[60]

An easily detectable marker of the shock syndrome is needed to help identify patients in the early phases. Serum assays for complement (C_{5a}), as an early marker have not lived up to expectations. However, another mediator, vasopressin, is currently being evaluated as a marker, since it has recently been shown to be elaborated in increased amounts by the CNS of dogs in early shock.[61]

Thus, the most important new direction of shock therapy in all age groups is earlier identification of the patient who is in the process of having the shock syndrome develop, because the primary cause of poor outcome is usually failure to institute therapy early enough. The identification of an early marker and the administration of specific antimediator drugs to infants and children in shock also holds promise for greater success in the treatment of shock in the future.

References

1. Stiehm R, Rich K: Recognition and management of shock in pediatric patients. Curr Probl Pediatr 3(4):3, 1973
2. Perkin R, Levin D: Shock in the pediatric patient, Part 1. J Pediatr 101:163, 1982
3. Warwick WJ, Ruttenberg HD, Quie PG: Sclerema neonatorum—a sign, not a disease. JAMA 1984:680, 1963
4. Sheldon R: Management of perinatal asphyxia and shock. Pediatr Ann 6:227, 1977
5. Johnson DG: Shock and its management. Pediatr Clin North Am 16:621, 1969
6. Shiller J: Shock in the newborn caused by transplacental hemorrhage from fetus to mother. Pediatrics 20:7, 1957
7. Becker A, Glass J: Twin-to-twin transfusion syndrome. Am J Dis Child 106:624, 1963
8. Hodes HL: Care of the critically ill child: Endotoxin shock. Pediatrics 44:248, 1969
9. Carr DB, Bergland R, Hamilton A et al: Endotoxin-stimulated opioid peptide secretion: Two secretory pools and feedback control in vivo. Science 217:845, 1982
10. Cohn J: Blood pressure measurement in shock. JAMA 199:118, 1967
11. Buck JR, Connors RH, Coon WW et al: Pulmonary embolism in children. J Pediatr Surg 16:385, 1981
12. Hughes WE, Hammond ML: Sclerema neonatorum. J Pediatr 32:676, 1948
13. Weil MH, Shubin H: Diagnosis and Treatment of Shock. Baltimore, Williams and Wilkins, 1967
14. Strodel W, Callaghan ML, Weintraub WH, Coran AG: The effect of various resuscitative regimens on hemorrhagic shock in puppies. J Pediatr Surg 12:809, 1977
15. Moss AJ, Adams FH: Problems of Blood Pressure in Childhood. Springfield, Illinois, Charles C Thomas, 1962

16. Moss AJ, Liebling W, Adams FH: The flush method for determining blood pressures in infants, Part II. Normal values during the first year of life. Pediatrics 21:950, 1958

17. Steier M: Neonatal and pediatric cardiovascular crisis. JAMA 235:1105, 1976

18. Coran AG: Mechanical support and monitoring procedures in the pediatric surgery patient. In Dudrick SJ et al (eds): Manual of Preoperative and Postoperative Care, 3rd ed. Philadelphia, WB Saunders, 1983

19. Weil MH, Shubin H, Rosoff L: Fluid repletion in circulatory shock: Central venous pressure and other practical guides. JAMA 192:668, 1965

20. Wilson JN, Grow JB, DeMong CV et al: Central venous pressure in optimal blood volume maintenance. Arch Surg 85:578, 1962

21. Raphaely RC: Shock. In Fleisher GR and Ludwig S (eds): Textbook of Pediatric Emergency Medicine. Baltimore, Williams and Wilkins, 1983

22. Callaghan ML, Weintraub WH, Coran AG: Assessment of thermodilution cardiac output in small subjects. J Pediatr Surg 11:269, 1976

23. Adamsons K Jr, Gandy GM, James LS: The influence of thermal factors upon oxygen consumption of the newborn infant. J Pediatr 66:508, 1965

24. Sonnenschein H: Endotoxin shock in infants and children. Med Trial Tech Q 19:134, 1973

25. Dechert R, Wesley J, Schafer L et al: Measurement of resting expenditure in premature infants. JPEN 8:100, 1984

26. Aubier M, Trippenbach T, Roussos C: Respiratory muscle fatigue during cardiogenic shock. J Appl Physiol 51:499, 1984

27. Bone R: Treatment of severe hypoxemia due to the adult respiratory distress syndrome. Arch Intern Med 140:85, 1980

28. Macklem PT: Respiratory muscles: The vital pump. Chest 78:753, 1980

29. Rowe M, Arango A: The choice of intravenous fluid in shock resuscitation. Pediatr Clin North Am 22:269, 1975

30. Shoemaker WC, Hauser CJ: Critique of crystalloid therapy in shock and shock lung. Crit Care Med 7:117, 1979

31. Benner J, Polley TZ, Strodel WE et al: Fluid resuscitation in live Eschericia coli shock in puppies. J Pediatr Surg 15:527, 1980

32. Moss G, Lowe RJ, Jilek J, Levine HD: Colloid or crystalloid in the resuscitation of hemorrhagic shock: A controlled clinical trial. Surgery 89:434, 1981

33. Greisman SE: Experimental gram-negative bacterial sepsis: Optimal methylprednisolone requirements for prevention of mortality not prevented by antibiotics. Proc Exp Biol Med 170:436, 1982

34. Russo-Marie F, Seillan C, Duval DL: Glucocorticoids as inhibitors of prostaglandin synthesis. Bull Eur Physiopathol Respir 17:587, 1981

35. Sheagren JN: Glucocorticoid therapy in the management of severe sepsis. In Sande MA and Rott RK (eds): Septic Shock: New Concepts of Pathophysiology and Treatment. New York, Churchill Livingstone, 1985

36. Hinshaw LB, Archer LT, Beller-Todd BK et al: Survival of primates in LD-100 septic shock following steroid/antiobiotic therapy. J Surg Res 2(8):151, 1980

37. Schumer W: Steroids in the treatment of clinical septic shock. Ann Surg 184:333, 1976

38. Connors R, Coran AG, Drongowski RA, Wesley JR: Combined fluid and corticosteroid therapy in septic shock in puppies. World J Surg 7:661, 1983

39. Hoffman SL, Punjabi NH, Kumala S et al: Reduction of mortality in chloramphenicol-treated severe typhoid fever by high-dose dexamethasone. N Engl J Med 310:82, 1984

40. Bone RC, Fisher CJ Jr, Clemmer TP et al: A controlled clinical trial of high-dose methylprednisolone in the treatment of severe sepsis and septic shock. N Engl J Med 317:654, 1987
41. Hinshaw L, Peduzzi P, Young E et al: Effect of high-dose glucocorticoid therapy on mortality in patients with clinical signs of systemic sepsis. N Engl J Med 317:659, 1987
42. Rowe MI, Buckner DM, Newmark S: The early diagnosis of gram negative septicemia in the pediatric surgical patient. Ann Surg 182:280, 1975
43. Behrendt D, Austen W: Patient Care in Cardiac Surgery, 3rd ed. Boston, Little, Brown and Co, 1980
44. Goldberg L: Drug therapy: Dopamine—clinical uses of endogenous catecholamine. N Engl J Med 291:707, 1974
45. Perkin R, Levin D: Shock in the pediatric patient, Part 2. J Pediatr 101:319, 1982
46. Driscoll D, Gillette P, McNamara D: The use of dopamine in children. J Pediatr 92:309, 1978
47. Albert SA, Shires GT III, Illner H, Shires GT: Effects of naloxone in hemorrhagic shock. Surg Gynecol Obstet 155:325, 1982
48. Brandt NJ, Terenius L, Jacobsen BB et al: Hyper-endorphin syndrome in a child with necrotizing encephalomyelopathy. N Engl J Med 303:914, 1980
49. Faden AI, Holaday JW: Experimental endotoxic shock: The pathophysiologic function of endorphin and treatment with opiate antagonists. J Infect Dis 142:229, 1980
50. Peters WP, Johnson MW, Friedman PA, Mitch WE: Pressor effect of naloxone in septic shock. Lancet 1:529, 1981
51. Zeigler E. McCutchan JA, Fierer J et al: Treatment of gram-negative bacteremia and shock with human antiserum to a mutant Eschericia coli. N Engl J Med 307:1225, 1982
52. Fletcher JR, Ramwell PW: Indomethacin treatment following baboon endotoxin shock improves survival. Adv Shock Res 4:103, 1980
53. Jacobs ER, Soulsby ME, Bone RC et al: Ibuprofen in canine endotoxic shock. J Clin Invest 70:536, 1982
54. Schmeling DJ, Drongowski RA, Coran AG: Protective effect of ibuprofen in a lethal septic shock model and relationship to oxidant injury. Circulatory Shock 24(4):239, 1988
55. Wise WC, Cook JA, Eller T, Halushka PV: Ibuprofen improves survival from endotoxin shock in the rat. J Pharmacol Exp Ther 215:160, 1980
56. Lefer AM, Tabas J, Smith EF: Salutary effects of prostacyclin in endotoxin shock. Pharmacol 21:206, 1980
57. Das JB, Indira JD, Philippart AI: End-tidal CO_2 and tissue pH in the monitoring of acid base changes: A composite technique for continuous, minimally-invasive monitoring. J Pediatr Surg 19:758, 1984
58. Morgan RA, Manning PB, Coran AG et al: Oxygen free radical activity during live E. coli septic shock in the dog. Circulatory Shock 25:319, 1988
59. Sheagren JN: Septic shock and corticosteroids. N Engl J Med 305:456, 1981
60. Bartlett RH et al: Extracorporeal circulation in neonatal respiratory failure: A prospective randomized study. Pediatrics 76:479, 1985
61. Cronenwett J, Sheagren JN: Personal Communication

CHAPTER 6

Recent Advances in Experimental Shock

G. Tom Shires, III

O ngoing major improvements in pre-hospital care, transport, initial resuscitation, and intensive care treatment have combined to increase survival in injured patients. Basic investigation characterizing the nature of cellular dysfunction in shock has led to major improvements in early care of the septic and injured patient. Initial resuscitation is now well developed, and has led not only to adequate therapy for routine injuries, but also to increasing salvage of the most severely injured. However, this improved early survival has resulted in a change in postresuscitation mortality, now most often the result of sepsis and generalized cell failure, characterized as multi-system organ failure syndrome. Three-fourths of patients with burn injury now die from septic complications, and multiple system organ failure, with its attendant high mortality, is most frequently associated with sepsis.

The next therapeutic frontier lies in understanding the underlying mechanisms of cellular derangement following injury. Increasingly, these effects appear to be mediated in large part by the host response to ischemia or tissue necrosis, bacteria and other infectious agents, and their products, including endotoxin. A variety of endogenous substances have recently been characterized as potential mediators of various shock states. Activation of complement and coagulation cascades, arachidonic acid metabolites, platelet-activating factor, and neutrophil activation with oxygen radical release have interrelated roles that lead ultimately to cell and tissue injury. In addition to these inflammatory mediators, lymphocyte-derived and macrophage/monocyte-derived protein hormones (collectively termed *lymphokines* and *monokines*) appear to play a central role. Translocation of bacteria from the intestinal lumen has recently been implicated as a source for the initial stimulus for this chain of events, secondary to a loss of gut mucosal integrity, bacterial overgrowth, or altered immunocompetence.

Bacterial endotoxin, or lipopolysaccharide (LPS), since its isolation in 1943,[1] has been the focus of numerous studies as the instigating factor in systemic response to sepsis. Infusion studies have characterized lethal tissue injury as the end result of altered metabolic and membrane functions. The acute inflammatory responses leading to organ dysfunction appear to be mediated not by LPS, but by humoral factors elaborated in response to endotoxemia. Diffuse intravascular coagulation is noted histologically, as is acute renal tubular necrosis and hemorrhagic congestion in the lung.[2]

Cachectin/tumor necrosis factor was first isolated from rabbit serum during active *Trypanosoma brucei* infection in 1980.[3] Further work purified the protein from LPS-stimulated macrophages.[4] A variety of cells are capable of producing cachectin following appropriate stimuli, including Kupffer cells, peritoneal and pulmonary macrophages, and circulating blood monocytes. Serum recovery of circulating cachectin is brief, reaching a peak within two hours following endotoxin infusion and falling below detection a few hours later.[5] Cachectin is distributed in liver, lung, kidney, and skin following injected radiolabeled doses.

Cachectin is an endogenous pyrogen that evokes a biphasic fever.[6] The early spike at one hour is the result of a direct hypothalamic PGE_2 effect, while the later peak appears to be mediated by interleukin-1. Studies of rats infused with recombinant human cachectin show severe systemic toxicity. Hypotension, acidosis, and shock culminated in death from respiratory arrest in a dose-dependent fashion.[7] Although there is a species-specific dose-response to the biologic effects of human cachectin, appropriate doses in other mammals result in similar systemic effects.[8] Histologic study reveals lesions similar to those described previously following endotoxemia, including pulmonary hemorrhage and congestion, ischemic necrosis of the bowel, and acute tubular necrosis. Interstitial edema is a frequent finding, which explains the hemoconcentration noted premortem.

These effects of cachectin administration may be blocked by prior passive immunization with monoclonal anticachectin antibodies. Of particular interest is a similar protective effect when baboons are protected from septic shock by pretreatment two hours before the infusion of a lethal dose of *E. coli* infusion.[9]

Thus, current evidence suggests that at the cellular level, cachectin may play a central role in mediating the response to systemic sepsis. Cachectin infusion mimics the clinical and histologic pattern seen experimentally in both bacteremia and endotoxemia, and anticachectin antibodies can prevent a substantial degree of these responses not only to cachectin infusion, but also to bacteremia.

Another endogenous inflammatory mediator is platelet-activating factor (PAF). This endogenous ether lipid is released from various cells, including platelets, leukocytes, and endothelial cells. Initial experimental work has shown that PAF fulfills the criteria of a mediator of endotoxemia in that infusion into experimental animals produces a picture similar to septic shock, including systemic hypotension, pulmonary hypertension, increased vascular permeability, and cardiac dysfunction.[10,11] In addition, PAF has been isolated in increased concentrations from rat blood and tissue following endotoxin challenge. Finally, specific PAF receptor antagonists improve survival and hemodynamics following either PAF or endotoxin infusion.[11]

Ongoing studies in our laboratory have examined the role of PAF in causing cardiac and hepatic dysfunction by using the PAF receptor antagonist CV-3988 during live *E. coli* challenge in the rat. CV-3988 has been shown to inhibit PAF-induced hypotension; thrombocytopenia and vascular permeability increases following endotoxin challenge.[12] Following the *E. coli* infusion, PAF blockade allowed maintenance of cardiac output, stroke volume, and the normal relationship between coronary blood flow and myocardial work when compared to vehicle-treated septic controls. Although isolated PAF infusion has decreased coronary blood flow experimentally, *E. coli* infusion in this study increased coronary blood flow over the PAF antagonist-treated rats. Thus, myocardial depression during bacteremia appears to be mediated by mechanisms other than the influence of unopposed PAF on coronary blood flow.[13]

E. coli infusion also depressed blood flow to the splanchnic viscera and kidney. The fractional organ flow decreased proportionally more in these organs, suggesting that a simple change in cardiac output is not responsible for gut ischemia. Again, PAF-infusion studies have documented gastrointestinal ischemia, as have cachectin-infusion studies. The ability to prevent cachectin induced bowel necrosis by pretreatment with PAF antagonist is of interest.[14] This supports the concept of complex interaction of many mediators in regulating splanchnic blood flow. Clinically, the use of multiple blocking or inhibiting agents directed at subsets of different pathways may be required to normalize blood flow during abnormal septic hemodynamic states. These limited examples demonstrate the difficulty in assessing the specific role of each mediator and the interaction between the various classes of lipid mediators and cytokines, *in vivo,* upon any single cell function.

Other studies have examined hepatocyte response to bacterial challenge by evaluating hepatic blood flow. These studies have validated the use of low-dose galactose clearance as a measure of effective hepatic blood flow (EHBF).[15] In the CV-3988 treated animals, a significant drop in EHBF during *E. coli* bacteremia could be prevented. Concomitantly, the resting transmembrane potential, which was depolarized in the untreated animals, was maintained in the PAF-blocked group.[16] Total hepatic flow as assessed by microsphere methodology was not depressed in those animals that did show a fall in EHBF. This suggests that localized ischemia with microsphere trapping in the absence of effective cell perfusion occurs during untreated bacteremia. The results of the present study support the hypothesis that bacteremia-induced PAF effects yield complex alterations in liver cell function, hepatic perfusion, and cardiovascular performance.

Recent studies have identified a variety of early impairments of the immune system following severe trauma. While these defects undoubtedly play a role in the evolution of the multiple-organ failure state, the search for the source of inoculum in late sepsis has focused upon the gut as a potential source. Although primary wounds, surgical incisions, and invasive monitoring devices may serve as portals of entry for exogenous contamination, clinical microbiology studies in traumatized and other immunocompromised patients are indicating endogenous flora as a major source of infection by means of poorly characterized routes of invasion.

Bacterial translocation, the passage of viable enteric bacteria from the intact gut into the lymphatic and systemic circulation, has been postulated for decades as a potential mechanism of systemic infection. Recent studies have documented in animal models its occurrence following thermal injury, hemorrhagic shock, and endotoxin administration.[17] Potential mechanisms include intestinal bacterial overgrowth, loss of integrity of the intestinal barrier, and altered host defenses.[18]

Our laboratory has recently focused on the interaction between burn shock and the effect of distant sepsis on bacterial translocation. Acute thermal injury clearly results in increased capillary permeability and hypovolemia as one cause of splanchnic hypoperfusion. In animals exposed to a 30 percent body surface area scald injury, gut flow decreased by 40 percent at 6 hours but returned to normal on postburn day one, three, and seven. A paired group immediately inoculated postburn with *Pseudomonas aeruginosa* had similar hemodynamics. However, bacterial translocation, which occurred in 80 percent of burned animals on day one, was limited to the mesenteric lymph nodes. Only the burn infected animals continued to have positive node cultures, and progressed to positive cultures of the blood and abdominal organs.

A subsequent study used angiotension converting enzyme inhibition to block the transient early postburn decrease in splanchnic perfusion. This decreased the incidence of positive mesenteric lymph node cultures from 75 percent to 20 percent, suggesting a role for ischemia and or reperfusion in the early translocation phenomenon. Finally, pretreatment with allopurinol had a similar effect on the early postburn translocation. However, this transient protective effect seen at postburn day one was not maintained in the burn infected animals. This group went on to develop not only positive node but also blood and solid organ cultures by postburn day four.

The exact pathophysiology of this prolonged and enhanced bacterial translocation following thermal injury and infection is unknown. Burn injury alone may allow initial translocation to occur by means of a loss of mucosal barrier integrity from postinjury ischemia. However, the absence of ongoing splanchnic blood flow impairment in either burn or burn infected models suggests other mechanisms may be important in the later postburn period. This data suggests that either altered host defenses that result from a response to a distant infection or a chronic mucosal injury mediated by other mechanisms, perhaps hormonal or cytokine-related, play a role in late translocation phenomena.

The above studies serve as brief introduction to the complex cellular changes being characterized in critical injury. The underlying mechanisms of cell derangement appear to be mediated in part by the host response. These alterations must be better defined to allow more specific interventions that may lead to improved clinical therapy. Host mediators, which developed as initial adaptive responses to severe injury, may now have maladaptive deleterious consequences in the evolutionarily brief setting of the resuscitated patient. Ongoing basic investigation into the variety of effects of these substances should eventually allow specific control of only the injurious component of an otherwise necessary humoral host response.

References

1. Shear MJ, Turner FC: Chemical treatment of tumors, Part V. Isolation of the hemorrhage-producing fraction for *Serratia marcescens (Bacillus prodigiosus)* culture filtrate. J Nat Cancer Inst 4:81–97, 1943

2. Balis JU, Rappaport ES, Gerber L et al: A primate model for prolonged endotoxin shock: Blood-vascular reactions and effects of glucocorticoids. Lab Invest 38:511–523, 1978

3. Rouzer CA, Cerami A: Hypertriglyceridemia associated with *Trypanosoma brucei* infections in rabbits: Role of effective triglyceride removal. Mol Biochem Parasitol 2:31–38, 1980

4. Beutler B, Mahoney J, LeTrang N et al: Purification of cachectin, a lipoprotein lipase-suppressing hormone secreted by endotoxin-induced RAW 264.7 cells. J Exp Med 161:984–995, 1985

5. Michie HR, Manogue KR, Spriggs DR et al: Detection of circulating tumor necrosis factor after endotoxin administration. N Engl J Med 318:1481–1481, 1988

6. Dinarello CA, Cannon JG, Wolff SM et al: Tumor necrosis factor (cachectin) is an endogenous pyrogen and induces production of interleukin-1. J Exp Med 163:1433–1450, 1986

7. Tracey KJ, Beutler B, Lowry SF et al: Shock and tissue injury induced by recombinant human cachectin. Science 234:470–474, 1986

8. Tracey KJ, Lowry SF, Fahey III TJ et al: Cachectin/tumor necrosis factor induces lethal shock and stress hormone responses in the dog. Surg Gynecol Obstet 164:415–422, 1987

9. Tracey KJ, Fong Y, Hess DG et al: Anti-cachectin/TNF monoclonal antibodies prevent septic shock during lethal bacteremia. Nature 330:662–664, 1987

10. Chang SW, Feddersen CO, Henson PM, Voelkel NF: Platelet-activating factor mediates hemodynamic changes and lung injury in endotoxin-treated rats. J Clin Invest 79:1498–1509, 1987

11. Doebber TW, Wu MS, Robbins JC et al: Platelet-activating factor (PAF) involvement in endotoxin-induced hypotension in rats. Studies with PAF-receptor antagonist kadsurenone. Biochem Biophys Res Commun 29:799–808, 1985

12. Terashita Z, Imura Y, Nishikawa K, Sumida S: Is platelet-activating factor (PAF) a mediator of endotoxin shock? Eur J Pharmacol 109:257–261, 1985

13. Minei JP, Shires III GT, Shires GT: PAF antagonist CV-3988 improves cardiac performance during live *E. coli* bacteremia. Circ Shock 24(4):253, 1988

14. X-M Sun, Hsueh W: Tumor necrosis factor (TNF)-induced bowel necrosis in rats: The role of platelet-activating factor (PAF). FASEB J 2:A414, 1988

15. Schirmer WJ, Townsend MC, Schirmer JM et al: Galactose elimination kinetics in sepsis. Arch Surg 122:349–354, 1987

16. Minei JP, Shires III GT, Jones DB, Shires GT: Platelet-activating factor antagonist CV-3988 prevents hepatocellular membrane dysfunction during live *E. coli* bacteremia. Surg Forum 39:24–26, 1988

17. Deitch EA, Berg RD: Endotoxin but not malnutrition promotes bacterial translocation of the gut flora in burned mice. J Trauma 27:161–169, 1987

18. Wilmore DW, Smith RJ, O'Dwyer ST et al: A central organ after surgical stress. Surg 104:917–923, 1988

19. Wells CL, Maddous MA, Simmons RL: Proposed mechanisms for the translocation of intestinal bacteria. Rev Inf Dis 10:958–979

CHAPTER 7

Role of Oxygen Radicals in Experimental Shock

Peter A. Ward, Hans P. Friedl, and Gerd O. Till

*T*he question of the involvement of oxygen radicals in the shock syndrome remains controversial and uncertain. Studies that use animal models of acute tissue injury, such as acute lung injury (e.g., following infusion of bacterial endotoxin), thermal trauma of skin, or ischemia-reperfusion injury of the small intestine, support the concept that whether derived from effector cells (e.g., neutrophils or macrophages) or target cells (e.g., vascular endothelial cells) oxygen radicals play a significant role in the pathogenesis of microvascular injury in lung, skin, gut, and other organs.[1] Most evidence of the involvement of oxygen radicals *in vivo* has been obtained by indirect means, such as monitoring the effects of antioxidant interventions and demonstrating the appearance of lipid peroxidation products in body fluids and tissues. However, it should be noted that newly established experimental approaches that allow direct measurement of oxidants *in vivo* appear to confirm the data that has been obtained by indirect means. For example, direct evidence that oxygen-derived free radicals contribute to post-ischemic myocardial injury has been obtained recently by employing electron paramagnetic resonance spectroscopy.[2] In this chapter, we will discuss briefly the nature of oxygen radicals and their sources, the role of cytokines in shock syndromes, the animal models of oxygen-radical-mediated tissue injury, and recent observations that suggest that histamine and xanthine oxidase may play an important role in oxidant-mediated acute tissue injury.

Oxygen Radicals

An *oxygen radical* is an unstable form of oxygen in which there is an unpaired electron in the outer orbit. This form of oxygen either will *oxidize* (shed an electron) or *reduce* (accept an electron) in order to dismute to a more stable condition. Irrespective of the source of oxygen radicals, the addition of electrons to molecular (fully oxidized) oxygen (O_2) results in a predictable sequence of products according to the following reactions.

1. $O_2 + e^-$ (electron) $\rightarrow O_2^-$ (superoxide anion)
2. $O_2^- + e^- \rightarrow H_2O_2$
3. $H_2O_2 + e^- + Fe^{2+} \rightarrow HO^{\bullet}$ (hydroxyl radical) $+ OH^- + Fe^{3+}$
4. $HO^{\bullet} + e^- \rightarrow H_2O$

As the reactions demonstrate, this sequential process of reduction of O_2 results in the formation of two oxygen radical species: O_2^- and $HO^{\bullet}$, the latter highly unstable. It is important to emphasize that $HO^{\bullet}$ generation requires the presence of a transition metal, especially ferrous ion (Fe^{2+}), which catalyzes the electron transfer. This is important because the presence of iron chelators may block the source of ferrous ion (which is ferric ion) and interfere with the formation of $HO^{\bullet}$. Finally, H_2O_2 can be converted enzymatically by myeloperoxidase in the presence of halide to another reactive species, hypochlorous acid (HOCl), hypobromous acid (HOBr), or hypoiodous acid (HOI). Evidence exists that HOCl can cause oxidative damage to chemical groups on cell membranes and also cause conversion of latent metallo enzymes of neutrophils (collagenase, gelatinase) to active enzyme species.[3]

Generation of O_2^-, H_2O_2, and $HO^{\bullet}$ occurs with several different enzymes: xanthine oxidase, present in some endothelial cells and in large amounts in the parenchyma of the liver and small bowel; NADPH oxidase, which is present in phagocytic cells (neutrophils, eosinophils, macrophages, and monocytes) and is the main oxygen-dependent pathway for microbicidal activity of phagocytic cells; the mitochondrial cytochrome pathway, which under normal conditions generates relatively little in the way of oxygen radicals; the cyclooxygenase pathway, present in a variety of cells and capable of generating small amounts of O_2^- when endoperoxide formation in arachidonic acid derivatives occurs; and the mixed function oxidases, which are present for the metabolism of xenobiotic compounds. Xanthine oxidase and NADPH oxidase are the two enzyme systems that appear closely associated with tissue injury related to the acute inflammatory reaction.

Cytokines

Cytokines represent an important class of biologically active polypeptides that have been incriminated in shock-like conditions. These products are protein-like in nature, varying in molecular weight from 6,000 to approximately 30,000, and are produced in large amounts by a variety of cells, especially stimulated macrophages and monocytes. Cytokines also have diverse biological functions, a diversity so great that the clinical terms adopted before clarification of cytokines' biological functions have often been misleading, and perhaps are nearly irrelevant (e.g., tumor necrosis factor [TNF]). The two cytokines that have been most extensively studied are TNF and interleukin-1 (IL-1). Although not necessary for our purpose, it should be stated that our focus will be on TNF-alpha and IL-1-beta, the subclassification reflecting the discovery of additional, closely related homologues of similar molecules (TNF-β and IL-α). The structure of these polypeptides and their broad biological activities have been described in detail elsewhere.[4,5]

TNF and IL-1 appear to be important in inflammatory conditions, shock-like syndromes, and a variety of other clinically relevant situations. These cytokines produce their biological effects through a diversity of mechanisms. Some of the most well described effects of TNF and IL-1 include their ability to directly stimulate neutrophils, monocytes, and macrophages, resulting in oxygen radical formation;[6,7] their ability to modify the phagocytic cell without producing a direct oxygen radical response, but causing the cells to be "primed" for enhanced oxygen radical generation in the presence of another stimulus; and their ability to induce protein synthesis in endothelial cells, resulting in the expression on the endothelial cell membrane of intercellular adhesion molecules (ICAMs). This last described effect has direct biological consequences. The adhesive interactions between neutrophils and endothelial cells are enhanced greatly by interaction between the ICAM and the complementary, adhesion-promoting molecule on the neutrophil, the CD11b/CD18 antigen, which is also known as complement receptor-3 (CR3) or MO1 antigen.[8] Not only is the adhesion interaction enhanced because of the cytokine-induced modification of the endothelial cell, but if neutrophils are activated, the oxygen products of the activated neutrophils can more effectively kill endothelial cells.[9] This observation may be relevant to clinical problems associated with infusion of TNF or interleukin-2 (which induces production of TNF).[10] In these situations, there is evidence that pulmonary microvasculature will sustain injury, as shown by the development of acute life-threatening pulmonary edema.[11]

There is only indirect evidence that the shock syndrome is related to a production of oxygen radicals. Markers of oxygen radical formation include the appearance of products of lipid peroxidation in plasma and evidence of disulfide formation in proteins (resulting from oxidation of sulfhydryl groups and their cross-linking). Evidence suggesting a link between the shock-like syndrome and cytokine formation (which may result in oxygen radical production) comes from the clinical ability to protect mice and subhuman primates from the lethal effects of bacterial endotoxin infusion (lipopolysaccharide) by pretreatment with antibody to TNF.[12,13] There is compelling evidence that TNF is responsible for the cardiovascular collapse, although there is no proof as yet that this is attributable to oxygen radicals. A more direct example of the link between oxygen radicals and tissue injury comes from recent evidence that ischemia of the small bowel in rats (from 80% reduction of blood flow to the superior mesenteric artery) followed by reperfusion results in evidence of injury to the small bowel and to the lung, as assessed by morphological changes and leakage of plasma proteins from the vascular compartment. This example of multi-organ failure is associated with the appearance in plasma of abruptly rising levels of TNF reperfusion and lung injury, which appears to be neutrophil mediated and oxygen radical dependent. Lung injury can be virtually abolished if animals are pretreated with antibody to TNF.[14] Similar observations of TNF-induced lung injury and its prevention by antibody against TNF have also been made in a rat model of hepatic ischemia-reperfusion.[15]

It has been suggested previously that in ischemia-reperfusion injury of the small bowel, tissue xanthine oxidase is activated and generates O_2^-, with a resulting influx of neutrophils. Most of the injury to the small bowel appears to be related to toxic oxygen products of the recruited neutrophils.[16] In the model of ischemia-perfusion injury to the small bowel, it may be the influx of neutrophils and the generation of toxic oxygen products that results in release of endotoxin from the human and/or the wall of the bowel, resulting in the rapid appearance of TNF, which in turn causes modification of pulmonary vascular endothelial cells and their injury by activated neutrophils.

Histamine and Xanthine Oxidase

Histamine has long been considered to play a pathophysiologic role in the shock syndrome.[17] Increased plasma and tissue levels of histamine have been reported recently in conscious and anesthetized dogs subjected to experimental hemorrhagic shock[18] and in a rat model of endotoxic shock.[19] On the other hand, studies in human patients demonstrated that blood histamine concentrations are not elevated during septic shock.[20] Whether histamine plays a role in the pathogenesis of the shock syndrome remains unclear. However, most investigators agree that histamine is not an important factor in the lethal outcome of septic or hemorrhagic shock.

Recent *in vivo* and *in vitro* studies in our laboratory have uncovered a potentially important link between histamine and the production by xanthine oxidase of toxic oxygen free radicals in ischemia and shock. Using a rat model system of shock lung, which is induced by systemic complement activation and is mediated by oxygen radicals,[21,22] we have observed concomitant rises in plasma of histamine and xanthine oxidase activity.[23] As shown in Figure 7-1, both plasma histamine and xanthine oxidase (XO) activity (but not xanthine dehydrogenase activity) signifi-

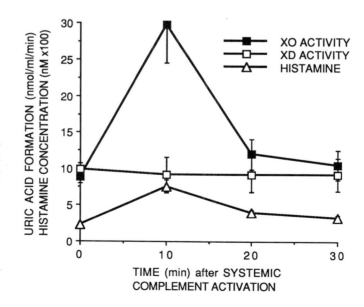

Figure 7-1. Appearance in plasma of increased levels of histamine and xanthine oxidase (XO) activity following systemic complement activation in rats. The activities of XO and xanthine dehydrogenase (XD) are expressed as nmol uric acid produced per ml of plasma per minute.

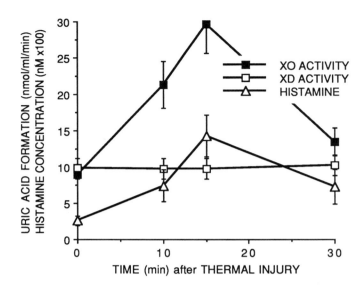

Figure 7-2. Thermal injury to the skin of rats resulting in a parallel rise in plasma histamine and xanthine oxidase (XO) activity. Xanthine dehydrogenase (XD) activity remains unchanged.

cantly increased with time, reaching peak values at 10 minutes after systemic complement activation. The increases in XO activity and histamine could be prevented by pretreatment of experimental animals with cromolyn, a mast cell stabilizer. The prevention of histamine release and the application of XO inhibitors significantly attenuated the oxygen radical-mediated acute pulmonary injury developed within 30 minutes after complement activation.

Additional evidence for a link between histamine and XO activity has been obtained in a rat model of thermal injury.[24] As depicted in Figure 7-2, a parallel rise in plasma XO activity and histamine could be observed peaking within 15 minutes after cutaneous burns. Again, plasma xanthine dehydrogenase (XD) activity remained unchanged. Pretreatment of experimental animals with cromolyn not only prevented the rise in histamine and XO‑activity, but also significantly attenuated the development of acute edema in the thermally injured skin.[24] The same degree of protection was seen when experimental animals were pretreated with XO inhibitors or scavengers of the hydroxyl radical,[25] suggesting a link between histamine levels, xanthine oxidase activity, and oxygen radical-mediated skin microvascular injury.

When normal rat plasma, which contains small amounts of XO as well as xanthine dehydrogenase (XD) activity, was incubated with varying concentrations of histamine in the presence of xanthine (substrate for XD/XO) and oxonate (to block uricase), a dose-dependent increase of XO (but not XD) activity was observed.[24] Maximal production of uric acid or superoxide anion by XO was seen at histamine levels of 1 uM. A similar enhancement by histamine was also observed when milk XO was employed. The mechanism of the interaction between histamine and XO to bring about catalytic enhancement of XO activity is presently unknown.

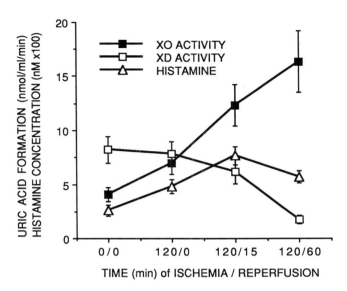

Figure 7-3. Intestinal ischemia-reperfusion in rats. Early appearance in plasma of XO activity paralleling the increase in plasma histamine levels. Beyond 15 minutes of reperfusion, the increase of XO activity results from a combination of histamine-induced XO enhancement and conversion of XD to XO as reflected by a significant decrease in XD activity.

Shock-related circulatory disorders are nearly always associated with the effects of ischemia. During shock states, vasoconstriction may occur in a variety of vascular beds, including such vital organs as lung, kidney, and gut. During reperfusion, XO-derived oxygen radicals are thought to play a crucial role in the development of cell and tissue injury.[16] Recent studies in our laboratory have provided evidence that histamine-enhanced XO activity also plays a role in ischemia-reperfusion injury. Employing a rat model of intestinal ischemia followed by reperfusion, we have observed that early increases in plasma XO activity following reperfusion were related to rises in plasma histamine levels (Figure 7-3). After about 15 minutes of reperfusion, conversion of XD to XO also contributed to the observed increase in XO activity.[26] Prevention of histamine release by pretreatment of experimental animals with cromolyn not only prevented the early rise in XO activity but also attenuated the ischemia-reperfusion injury. Similar observations of histamine-enhanced XO activity in plasma following ischemia reperfusion were also made in human patients undergoing upper extremity surgery under conditions of complete ischemia with tourniquet application.[27]

Conclusion

Despite significant advances in shock research and the description of a multitude of mediators thought to be involved in the development of shock-like syndromes, it is still unclear which mediators are important in the pathophysiology of shock. With regard to oxygen-derived free radicals, there is increasing experimental evidence to suggest that oxidants can cause injury to microvascular endothelial cells, which results in damage to the so-called shock organs. Antioxidant treatment not only decreases the amount of tissue damage and multiple organ failure, but also improves the survival rate of shock victims. The recently discovered connection between histamine and oxygen radical production by means of enhancement of xanthine oxidase activity may open up new avenues in the treatment and prevention of cell and tissue damage during ischemia and shock.

References

1. Fantone JC, Ward PA: Role of oxygen-derived free radicals and metabolites in leukocyte-dependent inflammatory reactions. Am J Pathol 107:395–418, 1982
2. Bolli R, Jeroudi MO, Patel BS et al: Direct evidence that oxygen-derived free radicals contribute to postischemic myocardial dysfunction in the intact dog. Proc Natl Acad Sci USA 86:4695–4699, 1989
3. Weiss SJ, Peppin GJ: Collagenolytic metalloenzymes of the human neutrophil characteristics, regulation and potential function in vivo. Biochem Pharmacol 35:3189–3197, 1986
4. Goeddel DV, Aggarwal BB, Gray PW et al: Tumor necrosis factors: Gene structure and biological activities. Cold Spring Harbor Symposia on Quantitative Biology, Cold Spring Harbor Laboratory 51:597–609, 1986
5. Dinarello CA: Interleukin-1: Amino acid sequences, multiple biological activities and comparison with tumor necrosis factor (cachectin). Year Immunol 2:68–89, 1986
6. Warren JS, Kunkel SL, Cunningham TW et al: Macrophage-derived cytokines amplify immune complex-triggered O_2^- responses by rat alveolar macrophages. Am J Pathol 130:489, 1988
7. Ozaki Y, Ohashi T, Niwa Y, Kume S: Effect of recombinant DNA-produced tumor necrosis factor on various parameters of neutrophil function. Inflammation 12:297–309, 1988
8. Marks RM, Todd III RF, Ward PA: Rapid induction of neutrophil–endothelial adhesion by endothelial complement fixation. Nature 339:314–317, 1989
9. Varani J, Fligiel SEG, Till GO et al: Pulmonary endothelial cell killing by human neutrophils: Possible involvement of hydroxyl radical. Lab Invest 53:656–663, 1985
10. Strieter RM, Remick DG, Lynch JP et al: Interleukin-2-induced tumor necrosis factor-α (TNF-α) gene expression in human alveolar macrophages and blood monocytes. Am Rev Respir Dis 139:335–342, 1989
11. Simpson SQ, Casey LC: Role of tumor necrosis factor in sepsis and acute lung injury. Crit Care Clin 5:27–47, 1989
12. Beutler B, Milsark IW, Cerami AC: Passive immunization against cachectin/tumor necrosis factor protects mice from lethal effect of endotoxin. Science 229:869–871, 1985
13. Tracey KJ, Fong Y, Hesse DG et al: Anti-cachectin/TNF monoclonal antibodies prevent septic shock during lethal bacteremia. Nature 330:662–664, 1987
14. Caty MG, Remick DG, Schmeling DJ et al: Evidence for endotoxin-related tumor necrosis factor (TNF) release in intestinal ischemia-reperfusion injury. Circ Shock 27:183A, 1989
15. Colletti LM, Burtch GD, Remick DG et al: Production of tumor necrosis factor alpha and the development of a pulmonary capillary injury following hepatic ischemia-reperfusion. Transplant Proc (in press)

16. Granger DN: Role of xanthine oxidase and granulocytes in ischemia-reperfusion injury. Am J Physiol 255:H1269–1275, 1988

17. Altura BM: Reticuloendothelial system function and histamine release in shock and trauma: Relationship to microcirculation. Klin Wochenschr 60:882–890, 1982

18. Nagy S, Nagy A, Adamicza A et al: Histamine level changes in the plasma and tissues in hemorrhagic shock. Circ Shock 18:227–239, 1986

19. Neugebauer E, Lorenz W, Beckurts T et al: Significance of histamine formation and release in the development of endotoxic shock: Proof of current concepts by randomized controlled studies in rats. Rev Infec Dis (Suppl 5):S585–S593, 1987

20. Jacobs R, Kaliner M, Shelhamer JH, Parrillo JE: Blood histamine concentrations are not elevated in humans with septic shock. Crit Care Med 17:30–35, 1989

21. Till GO, Johnson KJ, Kunkel R, Ward PA: Intravascular activation of complement and acute lung injury: Dependency on neutrophils and toxic oxygen metabolites. J Clin Invest 69:1126–1135, 1982

22. Ward PA, Till GO, Kunkel R, Beauchamp C: Evidence for role of hydroxyl radical in complement and neutrophil-dependent tissue injury. J Clin Invest 72:789–801, 1983

23. Till GO, Friedl HP, Guilds LS et al: Role of histamine in oxygen radical-mediated acute lung injury. FASEB J 3:A104, 1989

24. Friedl HP, Till GO, Trentz O, Ward PA: Role of histamine complement and xanthine oxidase in thermal injury of skin. Am J Pathol 1989 (in press)

25. Till Go, Guilds LS, Mahrougui M et al: Role of xanthine oxidase in thermal injury of skin. Am J Pathol 1989 (in press)

26. Caty MG, Schmeling DJ, Friedl HP et al: Histamine: A promoter of xanthine oxidase activity in intestinal ischemia-reperfusion. J Ped Surg (in press)

27. Friedl HP, Smith DJ, Thompson PD et al: Histamine and xanthine oxidase activity in a human model of ischemia reperfusion injury. Surg Forum (in press)

CHAPTER 8

Nutritional Support in Pediatric Trauma

John R. Wesley and Arnold G. Coran

*N*utritional support of a pediatric trauma victim is often a more complex therapeutic problem than nutritional support of an adult. In addition to the metabolic demands imposed by the traumatic event, special consideration must be
given to the pediatric patient because of smaller body size, highly variable fluid
requirements, rapid growth, and, in the newborn, the immaturity of certain organ
systems. These factors, plus the low caloric reserves of the young child, make adequate nutrition particularly important. Even a relatively short period of inadequate
nutrition can result in decreased host resistance, increased risk of infection, and
poor wound healing, which in turn contributes appreciably to morbidity and mortality. Although the nutritional requirements of teenagers do not differ significantly
from those of adults, the requirements of infants and young children are very different. This chapter focuses on nutritional requirements, and the procedures for
assessment and support of the pediatric age groups most often involved with
trauma: the toddler, young child, and teenager. Emphasis is placed on basic nutritional requirements, indications for initiating nutritional support, nutritional assessment and monitoring, and a summary of the important techniques for administration of enteral and parenteral nutrition.

Basic Nutritional Requirements

A young patient who is recovering from major trauma quickly uses readily available
glucose and glycogen stores, dips into fat stores, and parasitizes protein stores—
to the detriment of visceral and somatic muscle function and immune defenses.
Most otherwise healthy older children and teenagers can tolerate this form of energy "deficit-spending" for only five to seven days. If the patient then remains unable to eat or drink adequate amounts to supply ongoing energy needs, increased
muscular weakness and impaired host defenses begin to cause clinical problems
of their own. Infants and younger children have an even shorter time period dur-

ing which they can tolerate lack of nutritional support. Therefore, one of a physician's most important responsibilities is to estimate or measure the patient's nutritional requirements, provide correct nutritional support by the most efficient route, and monitor the effectiveness of the support. A knowledge of nutritional physiology is important to successfully establishing a daily caloric-protein budget.

Water

In infants, water makes up 70 to 75 percent of body weight, compared to 60 to 65 percent in adults. Therefore, the water requirements per unit of body weight are greater for infants and small children than for adults. The healthy infant consumes water at a daily rate of 10 to 15 percent of body weight, in contrast to only 2 to 4 percent by the teenager and adult. In circumstances of good health, only 0.5 to 3% of an infant's fluid intake is retained, with approximately 50 percent excreted through the kidneys, 3 to 10 percent lost through the gastrointestinal tract, and 40 to 50 percent insensible loss.

Calories

The caloric requirements for infants and children are outlined in Table 8-1. Energy requirements are often increased by periods of active growth and extreme physical activity. In addition to increased energy requirements caused by growth, major trauma or surgical stress increases the caloric requirements as follows: 12 percent increase for each degree of fever above 37°C, 20 to 30 percent increase with a major operation, 40 to 50 percent increase with severe sepsis, and 50 to 100 percent increase with major burns. In establishing a daily caloric budget for hospitalized patients, the physician should approximate the distribution of kilocalories according to that found in a well-balanced diet: protein, 15 percent; carbohydrate, 50 percent; and fat, 35 percent. In formula-fed or nursing infants, the values for carbohydrate and fat are reversed because of the increased fat requirement of a rapidly growing central nervous system.

Table 8-1. Estimated Protein and Calorie Requirements for Infants and Children

	Protein (gm/kg body weight)	Kilocalories (kcal/kg body weight)
0–1 years	2.0–3.5	90–120
1–7 years	2.0–2.5	75–90
7–12 years	2	60–75
12–18 years	1.5	30–60
›18 years	1	25–30

Carbohydrates

Carbohydrates are the most important immediate energy source, but their reserves in the body are the smallest in quantity. The total carbohydrate reserve in the average 70 kg man is only 2400 calories, with approximately equal distribution between the liver and skeletal muscle. Carbohydrate is stored primarily as glycogen and, in the infant, accounts for approximately 10 percent of body weight. Because the liver and muscle mass is proportionately much smaller in young children than in the adult, their carbohydrate reserve is significantly smaller. Glycogen is converted to glucose within the liver and is then metabolized throughout the body, either aerobically to carbon dioxide and water, (38 mols of APT/mol of glucose) or anaerobically to lactic acid (2 mols of ATP/mol of glucose). Aerobic metabolism of carbohydrates supplies 3.4 calories per gram (hydrous), requires 1 liter of oxygen for each 5 kilocalories produced, and gives off a volume of carbon dioxide equal to the volume of oxygen consumed for a respiratory quotient of 1 (RQ = ratio of CO_2 produced to O_2 consumed).

Fat

Fat is the major source of nonprotein calories for the human body, with reserves totaling 140,000 calories in the average 70 kg man. Because young children and rapidly growing adolescents frequently have less fatty tissue than adults, their energy stores are reduced proportionately. Fat is the most efficient energy source per unit weight, providing 9 kilocalories per gram and 4.7 kilocalories per liter of oxygen consumed, with an RQ of 0.7. This is the lowest RQ of the three energy sources and therefore results in the least amount of carbon dioxide and respiratory work per unit of energy produced. This is an important fact to consider in setting up a calorie budget for a patient with incipient respiratory failure or in a patient having difficulty weaning from a respirator.[1] Essential fatty acids (linoleic) must be supplied to the extent of at least 2 to 4 percent of daily administered kilocalories to avoid a deficiency syndrome characterized by hair loss; a dry, flaky, erthymetous skin rash; decreased platelet aggregation; and thrombocytopenia. In general, fat intake should not exceed 50 percent of the total caloric load because of the possibility of developing the fat overload syndrome.[2]

Protein

Protein makes up 13 percent of body weight in an infant, compared to 20 percent in the adult. Most of the proportional increase in body protein occurs during the first year of life, which is reflected in the major protein requirements based on the combined needs of maintenance and growth that exist during infancy. Protein provides 4.1 kilocalories per gram and 4.5 kilocalories for each liter of oxygen consumed, with an RQ of 0.8. Protein metabolism is most conveniently measured as nitrogen flux, and during trauma or critical stress, the rate of protein catabolism generally increases while intake stops, resulting in a condition commonly referred to as *negative nitrogen balance.*

Body protein is not intended as an intrinsic energy source because all body proteins are contained in structural elements whose integrity must be preserved for normal organ function, enzyme elaboration, and antibody production. Nevertheless, it appears that any traumatic event results in an obligatory catabolism of a variable amount of protein during the first 24 to 48 hours.[1] This protein breakdown is necessary to produce more glucose through the gluconeogenic pathway when carbohydrate stores have been exhausted. A negative nitrogen balance does not mean that protein synthesis stops or slows down; rather the synthesis of new cells, collagen, coagulation factors, inflammatory cells, antibodies, and a multitude of other biological proteins occurs at an accelerated rate during critical stress. Amino acids derived from the breakdown of muscle tissue or visceral proteins become the building blocks for protein in supplying host defense mechanisms and in healing tissues. A traumatic or surgical wound is a "privileged" site for approximately 14 days, during which time protein building blocks are diverted from other visceral and somatic sites in favor of wound healing. If extrinsic energy and protein sources have not been re-established after this period of time, the wound loses its privileged status and becomes a source for needed energy along with other protein matrices in the body. Left unchecked, this catabolism may lead to wound dehiscence and further potentially disastrous infectious complications.

A major goal of nutritional management is to provide an energy source so that endogenous proteins are not required for energy, and to supply exogenous proteins so that after a brief period of obligatory protein catabolism, all of the needs of protein synthesis can be met without breaking down the patient's own vital protein structures. In this regard, the amino acid composition of protein administered to infants and children is important in determining its nutritional value. Of the 20 amino acids identified in mammalian physiology, 9 are essential in infants and children; and 2 additional amino acids may be essential in the premature infant (Table 8-2). All of the essential amino acids must be present simultaneously in the diet for the formation of new lean body tissue. The absence of a single essential amino acid will result in a negative nitrogen and protein balance.

When a balanced energy source is provided early in the course of recovery,

Table 8-2. Essential Amino Acids

Valine	Phenylalanine
Leucine	Methionine
Isoleucine	Tryptophan
Threonine	Histidine*
Lysine	Tyrosine†
	Cystine†

*Essential only in infancy
†May be essential in the premature infant

somatic and visceral protein catabolism can be minimized, resulting in a "protein-sparing" effect. A number of clinical and experimental investigations have found that nitrogen sparing is achieved when the total nonprotein-calorie to gram-nitrogen ratio is 150–300:1.[3,4] Not only does the appropriate amount of administered fat and carbohydrate "spare" the continued breakdown of body protein for energy needs, but, after an initial period of obligatory protein breakdown, it also allows the administered intravenous or enteral protein to be laid down as new lean body mass.

A sufficient supply of carbohydrate appears to be the most important factor in achieving a protein-sparing effect. Hypocaloric infusions of glucose (5% dextrose in water or 5% dextrose in normal saline) are administered to provide the fluid requirements that prevent ketosis from fatty acid mobilization and help stave off some protein catabolism initially, but these are inadequate energy sources for even a short period of 2 to 3 days. Higher concentrations of glucose have proved effective, but must be administered by central venous infusion. When given by continuous drip with the appropriate amount of intravenous protein, they result in effective protein-sparing. However, as noted above, any energy source devoid of fat for 2 to 3 weeks may lead to the development of essential fatty acid deficiency, and also result in delayed or reduced development of the central nervous system. Because fat is such an efficient source of calories, clinicians have investigated using it as a sole source of energy and protein-sparing.[5–7] An elegant study by Brennan and colleagues showed that the protein-sparing effect was actually the result of the glycerol in which the lipid was suspended, plus the esterified glycerol in the triglyceride.[8] Other studies have shown that intravenous fat is protein-sparing both in children and adults.[3,7,9,10] Thus, fat given in disproportionately large quantities becomes a very expensive source of carbohydrate. The same can be said with respect to protein. Given alone in sufficient quantities, solutions of intravenous protein spare the host's lean body mass from being consumed for energy needs. But this occurs only because the intravenous protein is itself transaminated in the liver and broken down into a very expensive source of carbohydrate. Therefore, a balanced mixture of carbohydrate, fat, and protein is the most effective means of providing a patient's energy and protein repletion requirements while minimizing the catabolism of lean body mass. The exact balance will depend on the specific patient's needs. For example, an adult requires only enough fat to prevent essential fatty acid deficiency (2–10% of daily calories), while an infant requires much more because of the rapidly growing central nervous system and the need for nerve sheath myelinization.

Electrolytes, Vitamins, and Trace Elements

The administration of a well-balanced nutritional regimen is dependent on careful attention to detail, and a check list is useful to ensure that no important step is omitted. The major components—carbohydrate, fat, and protein—require the presence of vitamin catalysts and trace element cofactors to drive the metabolic machinery and achieve the desired anabolic effect. The absence or deficiency of

Table 8-3. Ranges for Electrolyte Supplements Recommended for Pediatric and Adolescent (Adult) Patients on TPN

Electrolyte	Infant Range (< 10 Kg)	Pediatric Range (10–30 Kg)	Adolescent Range (> 30 Kg)
Sodium	2–4 mEq/kg/day	20–150 mEq/day	60–150 mEq/day
Potassium	2–4 mEq/kg/day	20–240 mEq/day	90–240 mEq/day
Calcium	0.5–3 mEq/kg/day	5–20 mEq/day	10–15 mEq/day
Phosphorus	0.5–1 mmol/kg/day	6–50 mmol/day	30–50 mmol/day
Magnesium	0.5–1 mEq/kg/day	4–24 mEq/day	8–24 mEq/day
Chloride	4–12 mEq/kg/day	20–150 mEq/day	60–150 mEq/day
Acetate	2–8 mEq/kg/day	20–120 mEq/day	80–120 mEq/day

even one small component may result in failure of an otherwise carefully designed nutritional program. For example, attention must be given to provide an adequate supply of daily electrolytes, keeping in mind that a patient uses potassium, calcium, magnesium, and phosphorus in increased amounts during tissue anabolism (Table 8-3). Calcium and phosphorus are also important because of the rapid skeletal growth-rate of a young child. Likewise, the infant and young child require more vitamins per kilogram of body weight than the adult, and a hypermetabolic patient will catabolize vitamins more rapidly than normal. Although fat soluble vitamin (A,D,K, and E) stores are plentiful and deficiencies tend to develop slowly in an otherwise healthy patient, water-soluble vitamins (B, C, and folic acid) must be replenished frequently, and the critically ill trauma patient may reach a deficiency state in a relatively short time. In addition, there is some evidence that high doses of vitamins A and C may be beneficial to patients with injuries.[11] A specially convened American Medical Association panel recently published recommendations for vitamin dosages with parenteral nutrition for adults and children (Table 8-4).[12]

Table 8-4. Daily Vitamin Supplements Recommended for Pediatric and Adolescent (Adult) Patients on TPN (According to AMA Guidelines)

Vitamin	Pediatric Amount/Day	Adolescent (Adult) Amount/Day
Ascorbic acid	80 mg	100 gm
Vitamin A	2300 IU	3300 IU
Vitamin D	400 IU	200 IU
Thiamine HCL (B_1)	1.2 mg	3 mg
Riboflavin (B_2)	1.4 mg	3.6 mg
Pyridoxine HCL (B_6)	1.0 mg	4 mg
Niacinamide	17 mg	40 mg
Pantothenic acid	5 mg	15 mg
Vitamin E	7 IU	1 IU
Biotin	20 μg	60 μg
Folic acid	140 μg	400 μg
Cyanocobalamin (B_{12})	1 μg	5 μg
Phytonadione (K_1)	200 μg	1 mg

Table 8-5. Daily Trace Element Supplements Recommended for Pediatric and Adolescent (Adult) Patients Receiving TPN

Element	Pediatric Amount (mcg)	Adolescent (Adult) Amount (mcg)
Copper (sulfate)	20	1
Zinc (sulfate)	300	5
Manganese (sulfate)	10	0.5
Chromium (chloride)	0.2	0.010
Selenium (selenious acid)	1.2	0.060

Trace elements are also important—zinc, copper, fluoride, chromium, manganese, and selenium have well known metabolic functions. Silicon, boron, nickel, aluminum, arsenic, tin, molybdenum, vanadium, and strontium are also required by the body, but their specific metabolic functions and the amounts needed have not been defined. In the early days of total parenteral nutrition, trace element deficiencies were seldom seen in patients who received protein hydrolysate because there existed a myriad of trace elements in the relatively impure biological protein mixture. Because of patient allergic reactions to the antigens in these biologic protein solutions, synthetic amino acids were developed, which are largely free of trace element "contaminants." This has necessitated in turn the addition of trace elements to TPN solutions, and we expect that it will not be long before additional trace elements, such as molybdenum and nickel, will be added to the list in Table 8-5.[13]

Nutritional Assessment and Monitoring

Assessment of nutritional requirements is an important part of the total evaluation of any seriously injured patient. Usually, a severely malnourished patient is easily recognized, even without anthropometric measurements and serum chemistries. However, patients in a state of moderate malnutrition are frequently a challenge to the physician's diagnostic skills. The first important step in providing proper nutritional therapy is early identification of patients who are at risk of progressing to severe nutritional depletion. Fortunately, most injured pediatric patients are reasonably well-nourished at the time of their accident, and nutritional support is preventive and supportive for the anticipated stress of the traumatic event, recovery process, and ongoing growth requirements, rather than therapeutic for pre-existing chronic deficiencies. Establishing simple baseline nutritional measures, such as height, weight, and head circumference, albumin, and total protein, provides direction for nutritional management. Traumatized patients who, through delay or oversight, slip into a state of malnutrition will develop impaired wound healing, compromised immune status, and increased morbidity and mortality. A complete nutritional assessment should include evaluation of risk factors, diet history, clinical examination (including basic anthropometric measurements and laboratory data), energy requirements, and, if available, indirect calorimetry. A discussion of basic anthropometrics can be found in standard textbooks and manuals of nutrition support, and will not be covered further in this discussion.[14]

The initial traumatic event is the obvious focal point for evaluation of risk factors. Large open wounds indicate the risk for protracted nutrient losses and increased metabolic needs. Similarly, the presence of extensive burns, blunt trauma, and the onset of fever indicate increased metabolic requirements. Recent loss of 10 percent or more of usual body weight, or the anticipation of nothing by mouth for more than 7 days on simple intravenous solutions, is an indication to start formal nutritional support. Changes in taste, appetite, prior consumption of a special diet, or poor intake prior to the traumatic event may indicate a significantly altered nutritional status. The clinical examination is very important in assessing the patient's nutritional state and potential need for nutritional intervention. Obviously, the assessment of vascular and gastrointestinal injuries have a direct bearing on the type and form of nutritional support that will be required. An important question in every instance is whether or not the gastrointestinal tract will be functional in 24 to 48 hours. A spinal cord injury or large retroperitoneal hematoma, for example, would be expected to lead to a prolonged ileus, and parenteral nutrition would be expected to be needed during the recovery period.

Assessment Indices

Because every molecule of protein in the body performs a vital function, and because protein is not stored in the body, protein depletion indicates nutritional impairment. The patient's protein status directly affects the ability to respond to stress, especially when fat or glycogen stores are also depleted. Therefore, nutritional assessment focuses on the protein compartments, both somatic (muscle) and visceral (all other proteins). Several indices may be measured for each compartment. Examples are weight, triceps skin fold, mid-arm muscle circumference, and creatinine height index for the somatic compartment, and serum albumin, transferrin, total lymphocyte count, and skin test reactivity for the visceral compartment. Because no single test or measurement adequately defines a patient's nutritional status, reliance on a single factor is inappropriate. Individual serum chemistries, however, are useful in noting potential toxicities or deficits, and trends observed are quite useful in assessing overall nutritional status. Every patient undergo need not undergo all available tests. However, every patient should have a daily weight recorded, as this is one of the most easily obtained and useful indicators of nutritional status. Weight loss often reflects the use of body protein (i.e., muscle and organ tissue) as a metabolic fuel, which occurs quickly when caloric intake in a traumatized patient is severely restricted. The patient's current weight should be used in conjunction with his or her usual weight, recent weight changes, and ideal weight for height. For accuracy, the patient should be weighed at the same time each day, on the same scale, in the same clothing, and by the same nurse.

Measuring a patient's nitrogen balance is a useful means of determining daily nitrogen requirements as well as the effectiveness of ongoing nutritional therapy. Accurate and rapid measurements of substances containing chemically bound nitrogen can be obtained by means of the 703C Chemoluminescent Nitrogen System.* Gaseous, liquid, or solid samples may be readily analyzed in less than one minute. The goal for growth or repair is a daily positive balance of 4 to 6 grams in the adolescent or adult, and proportionately less in the infant and small child. A 24-hour urine collection is necessary, which makes the balance study somewhat difficult to obtain. Protein intake, whether enteral or parenteral, needs to be accurately recorded.

Energy requirements for traumatized patients can be calculated either by the use of nomograms or by respirometry and indirect calorimetry. Nomograms usually provide an estimated basal energy expenditure (BEE) based on age, height, and weight, and provide factors for computation of energy expended as the result of additional stress, such as postoperative recovery, multiple trauma, fever, and severe infection. These are readily found in standard textbooks and manuals.[14,15]

Numerous studies of nutritional requirements during health and disease have been based on estimated energy expenditure. Actual measurement, however, is now more available and more accurate, and is becoming an important aspect of critical care management. The most commonly used method of measurement is *indirect calorimetry*. In this method, the amount of oxygen absorbed across the lung is assumed to be exactly equal to the amount of oxygen consumed in metabolic processes. This is the basic assumption of the Fick equation and is the reason why oxygen consumption is a valid measure of metabolism, even in patients with abnormal lung function.

We have recently developed a method of closed-circuit, water-sealed indirect calorimetry for infants who are breathing spontaneously, which enables measurement of oxygen consumption, carbon dioxide production, and calculation of caloric expenditure using the Weir equation.[16] The measurements obtained have demonstrated a much wider range of energy expenditure for infants of similar weight and gestational age than that calculated by nomograms and tables.[17] We have found that commonly used nomograms may underestimate energy expenditure by as much as 70 percent.[18]

Although indirect calorimetry is easy to perform in patients who are not intubated and are breathing spontaneously, many critically ill patients are intubated and on mechanical ventilators, which complicates the technique of measuring oxygen consumption and carbon dioxide production.[19] We have recently tested a miniature indirect calorimetry device that can be interposed between the patient's pressure-limited respirator and endotracheal tube, and that greatly simplifies the problem of measuring oxygen consumption for infants maintained on pressure-limited respirators.[6]

The above methods of nutritional assessment are used to classify the nutri-

---

*Antek Instruments, Houston, Texas

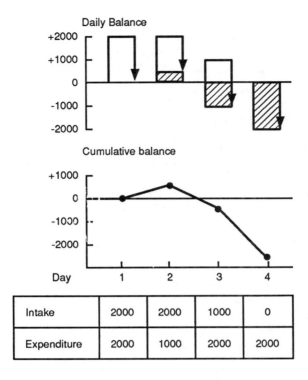

	Day 1	Day 2	Day 3	Day 4
Intake	2000	2000	1000	0
Expenditure	2000	1000	2000	2000

Figure 8-1. Measurement of Cumulative Energy Balance

tional status of patients at the time of injury, operation, or critical illness. Baker and collegues have shown that a careful clinical examination is as accurate as more complex and expensive laboratory and anthropometric measurements in identifying malnutrition in stressed patients.[20] In another excellent study, Forse and Shizgal measured body cell mass (the "gold standard" for measurement of nutritional status) and found that the depleted state could not be detected reliably based on weight–height ratio, triceps skin fold, mid-arm circumference, albumin, total protein, hand strength, or creatinine–height ratio.[21] Actual measurement or estimation of metabolic rate is the best method of following nutritional status in a critically ill patient.

In summary, daily energy requirements should be estimated at the very least, and, at best, metabolic rate and cumulative caloric balance should be measured daily. A diagrammatic representation of such balance measurement is shown in Figure 8-1. The intake is plotted upward from the baseline, and the output or caloric expenditure is plotted downward from the top of the intake line. Therefore, positive balance will appear as deviation above the baseline and negative balance as deviation below the baseline. By totalling the daily positive or negative balance in a running fashion, the cumulative caloric balance can be determined. Bartlett and colleagues have determined that acutely ill adult patients with caloric deficits greater than 10,000 calories have a much higher mortality than patients with positive caloric balance.[22] Similar studies have yet to be done in infants and children.

Administration of Enteral and Parenteral Nutrition

A pediatric patient who is healthy at the time of accidental injury or major surgery can sustain a five to seven day interval without significant energy intake and have no serious systemic consequences provided that adequate nutritional support is initiated thereafter. However, it is easier to preserve lean body mass than to make up for its catabolism and deficiency. Therefore, nutritional support should be started as soon as practicable after trauma or major surgery. The type of nutritional support depends on the form and extent of stress affecting the individual child.

With respect to physiologic efficiency and the economy of administration, enteral feedings are preferable and should be the first choice in patients with adequate function of the gastrointestinal tract.[23,24] The rapid development of modern high technology has made enteral feeding possible in most traumatized patients. Enteral feedings can provide protein, with glutamine and other special nutrients, equivalent to or better than that supplied by total parenteral nutrition and can be furnished at a greatly reduced cost. Nasoenteric tube feedings are appropriate for most situations in which the ability for oral feeding is slow to return.[25] Gastrostomy is most useful for long-term enteral feeding and, when appropriate, catheter jejunostomy has the advantage of providing a route for enteral support during the recovery phase of postoperative ileus, and at reduced risk of aspiration because of infusion beyond the pylorus.[26,27] The use of fluoroscopy and flexible endoscopy aids in the placement of feeding tubes at various sites in the gastrointestinal tract, often avoiding the need for additional surgery, and hastening the transition from parenteral nutrition to full enteral support.[28]

Because fewer children than previously undergo abdominal exploration for blunt trauma, the decision to place a feeding gastrostomy or catheter jejunostomy is usually a primary one, made later in the course of the patient's recovery. When considering operative placement of a feeding gastrostomy, the physician should always evaluate the patient for gastroesophageal reflux, which, if present, frequently will be worsened by the addition of the gastrostomy tube.[29] This is especially important in the case of brain-damaged children, for whom uncontrolled reflux is particularly dangerous.[30] Pre-operative evaluation is indicated, and generally consists of a barium swallow and limited upper-gastrointestinal series, followed by a 24-hour *p*H monitoring. If these tests are positive for reflux, then a fundoplication should be performed at the time of gastrostomy. If poor gastric motility and slow emptying are also documented, then a pyloroplasty should be added to the procedure. Recently, the percutaneous endoscopy technique for placing a feeding gastrostomy without the need for laparotomy has been extended to children.[31,32] It is performed with the aid of a flexible fiberoptic endoscope, and, in experienced hands, has proven safe and effective for selected patients.

When an abdominal exploration is required during early treatment of the traumatized pediatric patient, catheter jejunostomy reportedly has provided an early and relatively safe postoperative route for enteral nutrition.[33] However, we have preferred a combination of early parenteral nutrition followed by nasogastric tube feedings later if necessary. Alternatively, when we have preferred jejunal feedings because of gastroesophageal reflux or poor gastric motility, we have placed a jejunal tube by means of a previously placed Stamm gastrostomy. The jejunal tube can be inserted through the gastrostomy stoma, with accurate placement of the tip under fluoroscopy, or with the aid of flexible endoscopy.[34]

Total Parenteral Nutrition

If the nutritionally compromised trauma patient is unable to accept or absorb enteral feedings, TPN is required. In infants and small children, TPN is indicated if there is inadequate nutrition for four or five days. In older children and adults, the tolerable period of inadequate nutrition may be longer, depending upon the nutritional status of the patient before the traumatic event. The benefits of TPN for reducing the risks of malnutrition must be weighed against the risks of serious complications, especially sepsis.

TPN can be administered by peripheral vein, although this route is sometimes limited by considerations of the high osmolality of the solution and the large volumes necessary to achieve adequate caloric support. In infants and small children, the external jugular, inferior thyroid, facial, and cephalic veins can be used for central venous access through the appropriate neck incision. A silastic catheter is preferred because of its flexibility and low thrombogenicity. Recently, the greater saphenous vein has been used successfully in children as an access site for inferior vena cava infusion, and can also be used in the adolescent when no other access site is available.[35] The recent development of miniature "peel-away" sheaths has enabled the percutaneous introduction of silastic catheters. The infraclavicular approach is the preferred route in older children and young adults, both because of the technical ease of insertion and because of patient comfort. A specific protocol should be followed at the time of insertion to to help ensure successful parenteral nutrition from the technical standpoint.[14] Parenteral nutrition is never an emergency; and, therefore, catheter insertion should be done under well-controlled conditions. Insertion of a central line for parenteral nutrition is a surgical procedure and requires the use of strict aseptic technique. After insertion, the site should be dressed using a standard dressing protocol.[14] The keys to catheter longevity are sterility of the catheter–skin junction and having an occlusive dressing in place at all times. A chest roentogram should be obtained immediately after placement of the central line to ascertain that it is in the correct position, prior to initiating infusion of the parenteral nutrition.

The composition of TPN solutions, protocols for administration and methods of monitoring are very important, and have been detailed in other textbooks and manuals.[14,15] Similarly, the technical, septic, and metabolic complications of intravenous nutritional support are well known and must be continually guarded against.[14] Careful attention to the details of patient care, indicating the team approach to managing nutritional support, will help obtain a successful outcome.[36]

Finally, the process of transition from parenteral back to oral-enteral nutrition is very important, and often difficult. If not well managed, the patient may lose a hard-earned nutritional advantage. Although it is important that nearly full caloric requirements be supplied before parenteral support is discontinued, it is often necessary to cut back by as much as half of the daily amount of parenteral nutrition to stimulate a patient's appetite and desire to eat. Bland clear liquids are often the first foods offered, and are barely acceptable to most patients. The early use of more appetizing food, such as popsicles, hard candy, commercial lactose-free formulas, cookies, and eggnog, should be encouraged. Accurate calorie counts are important to measure the patient's progress, but are notoriously difficult to obtain in the hospital. If possible, the patient or family member should be put in charge of this task and be impressed with its importance. A side benefit of this task is the positive effect it frequently has on the patient's or parents' pyschological sense of well-being.

References

1. Jeejeeboy KN, Marliss EB: Energy supply and total parenteral nutrition. In Fischer JE (ed): Surgical Nutrition, p 645. Boston, Little, Brown & Co, 1983

2. Adamkin DH, Gelke KN, Andrews BF: Fat emulsion and hypertriglyceridemia. JPEN 8:563, 1984

3. Benner JW, Coran AG, Weintraub WH, et al: The importance of different calorie sources in the intravenous nutrition of infants and children. Surgery 86:429, 1979

4. Kinney JM: Energy requirements for parenteral nutrition. In Fischer JE (ed): Total Parenteral Nutrition, p 135. Boston, Little, Brown & Co, 1976

5. Gazzaniga AB, Bartlett RH, Shobe JB: Nitrogen balance in patients receiving either fat or carbohydrate for total intravenous nutrition. Ann Surg 182:163, 1975

6. Heiss K, Hirschl R, Cilley R, et al: Measuring infant metabolism: Design and testing of a miniature gas exchange monitor. J Pediatr Surg 23:543, 1988

7. Jeejeebhoy KN, Anderson GH, Nakhooda AF, et al: Metabolic studies in total parenteral nutrition with lipid in man: Comparison with glucose. J Clin Invest 57:125, 1976

8. Brennan MF, Fitzpatrick GF, Cohen KH, et al: Glycerol: Major contributor to the short-term protein sparing effect of fat emulsions in normal man. Ann Surg 182:836, 1975

9. Coran AG: The long-term intravenous feeding of infants using peripheral veins. J Pediatr Surg 8:801, 1973

10. Coran AG: Total intravenous feeding of infants and children without the use of central venous catheter. Ann Surg 179:445, 1974

11. Gann DS, Robinson HB: Salt, water, and vitamins. In: ACS Manual of Surgical Nutrition, p 73. Philadelphia, WB Saunders, 1973

12. Multivitamin preparations for parenteral use: A statement by the Nutrition Advisory Group, American Medical Association. JPEN 3:258, 1979

13. Shils ME: AMA Department of Foods and Nutrition: Guidelines for essential trace element preparations for parenteral use: A statement by an expert panel. JAMA 241:2051, 1979

14. Wesley JR, Khalidi N, Faubion WC et al: The University of Michigan Hospitals' Parenteral and Enteral Nutrition Manual, ed 5. North Chicago, Illinois, Abbott Laboratories, Hospital Products Division, 1988

15. Kerner JA: Manual of pediatric parenteral nutrition. New York, John Wiley & Sons, 1983

16. Dechert RE, Wesley JR, Schafer LE et al: A water-sealed indirect calorimeter for measurement of oxygen consumption (VO_2), carbon dioxide production (VCO_2), and energy expenditure in infants. J Parent Enteral Nutr 12:256, 1988

17. Dechert R., Wesley J.R., Schafer L., et al: Comparison of oxygen consumption (VO_2), carbon dioxide production (VCO_2) and resting energy expenditure (REE) in premature and full-term infants. J Pediatr Surg 20:765, 1985

18. Mendeloff E, Wesley JR, Deckert RE et al: Comparison of measured resting energy expenditure (REE) versus estimated energy expenditure (EEE) in infants. JPEN 10 (Suppl):65, 1986

19. Wesley JR, Tse Y, Dechert R: Indirect calorimetry on mechanically ventilated rabbits. European Society of Parenteral and Enteral Nutrition, Paris, September 17, 1987

20. Baker JP, Detsky AS, Wesson D et al: Nutritional assessment: A comparison of clinical judgement and objective measurements. N Engl J Med 306:969, 1982

21. Forse RA, Shizgal HM: The assessment of malnutrition. Surgery 88:17, 1980

22. Bartlett RH, Dechert RE, Mault JR et al: Measurement of metabolism in multiple organ failure. Surgery 92:771, 1982

23. Balistreri WF, Farrell MK (eds): Enteral Feeding: Scientific Basis and Clinical Applications. Report of the Ninety-Fourth Ross Conference on Pediatric Research. Columbus, Ohio, Ross Laboratories, 1988

24. Randall HT, Bauer RH, Hickey MD et al: Early postoperative feeding (symposium). Contemp Surg 30:97, 1987

25. Rombeau JL, Jacobs DO: Nasoenteric tube feeding. In Rombeau JL, Caldwell MD (eds): Enteral and Tube Feeding, p 261. Philadelphia, WB Saunders, 1984

26. Gallagher MW, Tyson KRT, Ashcraft KW: Gastrostomy in pediatric patients: An analysis of complications and techniques. Surgery 74:536, 1973

27. Rombeau JL, Barot LR, Low DW et al: Feeding by tube enterostomy. In Rombeau JL, and Caldwell MD (eds): Enteral and Tube Feeding, p 274. Philadelphia, WB Saunders, 1984

28. Mclean GK: Radiologic technique of gastrointestinal intubation. In Rombeau JL, Caldwell MD (eds): Enteral and Tube Feeding, p 240. Philadelphia, WB Saunders, 1984

29. Canal DF, Vane DW, Seiichi G: Reduction of lower esophageal sphincter pressure with Stamm gastrostomy. J Pediatr Surg 22:54, 1987

30. Wesley JR, Coran AG, Sarahan TM et al: The need for evaluation of gastroesophageal reflux in brain-damaged children referred for feeding gastrostomy. J Pediatr Surg 16:866, 1981

31. Behkov KJ, Kazlow PG, Waye JD et al: Percutaneous endoscopic gastrostomies in children. Pediatrics 177:248, 1986

32. Gauderer ML, Ponsky JL, Izant RJ: Gastrostomy without laparotomy: A percutaneous endoscopic technique. J Pediatr Surg 15:872, 1980

33. Page CP, Carlton PK, Andrassy RJ et al: Safe, cost-effective post operative nutrition: Defined formula diet via needle catheter jejunostomy. Am J Surg 138:939, 1979

34. Mukherjee D, Emmens RE, Putnam TC: Nonoperative conversion of gastrostomy to feeding jejunostomy in children and adults. Surg Gynecol Obstet 154:881, 1982

35. Fonkalsrud EW, Berquist W, Burke M et al: Long-term hyperalimentation in children through saphenous central venous catheterization. Am J Surg 143:209, 1982

36. Faubion WC, Wesley JR, Khalidi N, Silva J: Total parenteral nutrition catheter sepsis: Impact of the team approach. JPEN 10:642, 1986

CHAPTER 9

Airway and Thoracic Injuries

James A. O'Neill, Jr.

E ighty five to ninety percent of injuries in childhood are the result of blunt forces and the remainder are from penetrating trauma.[1] It is estimated that 25 percent of the deaths resulting from trauma in childhood are related to cardiothoracic injuries, while the rate may be as high as 50 percent in adults.[2] This statistic adds emphasis to the point that injuries to the thorax and airway are of the highest priority in early management of the injured child because they are most likely to be responsible for early mortality. The overall mortality associated with cardiothoracic trauma in children is between 7 and 15 percent.[1,3] The younger the child, the higher the chance of mortality. If other organ systems are severely injured in addition to the thorax and airway, overall mortality incidence has been reported as high as 60 percent.[2,4]

Anatomic and Physiologic Considerations Specific to the Child

The larynx and trachea are much smaller in children (compared with adults) so obstruction by mucus, blood, vomitus, or other debris such as teeth is far more likely to occur in children. Additionally, because the ratio of smooth muscle to cartilage is greater in childhood than at any other time in life, bronchospasm related to the presence of foreign material in the tracheobronchial tree is more frequent in pediatric age patients.[5] The distance from the mouth to the carina is directly proportional to body weight. Because in young children this distance is relatively short, the danger of bronchial rather than tracheal placement of an endotracheal tube is a problem frequently encountered.[6]

Pliability of the chest wall is perhaps the most characteristic feature of the pediatric thorax, and it is well known that infants and children may sustain lethal internal thoracic injuries without any evidence of rib fractures.[1] In fact, it has been reported that mortality from intrathoracic injuries is higher in those pediatric patients with no rib fractures.[4] However, this may be a consideration of age. At least it points out the error of a physician assuming that intrathoracic injury is either minor or absent simply because no rib fractures are identified. Another pediatric age group consideration that is related to flexibility is mediastinal movement. In adults the mediastinum is relatively fixed, but this is not the case in children, and pneumothorax or hemopneumothorax under tension may result in marked shifts of the mediastinum with impairment of pulmonary expansion on the opposite side, as well as angulation of the cavae with impaired venous return to the heart. In this regard, adolescents' physiological response is more like that of adults.

Children tend to hyperventilate in response to trauma and have an accentuated tendency to swallow air. Gastric dilatation in the child produces more marked pathophysiologic consequences than those seen in adults and are related to impairment of diaphragmatic movement as well as vena caval compression impairing venous return.

Finally, children have varying respiratory rates related to their age; this must be kept in mind when artificial ventilatory support is required.[7]

Airway Injuries

Initial evaluation of a patient with a thoracic injury or an airway injury in the neck is the same for all injured patients. This involves a rapid initial survey of the entire body with priority attention directed at establishing an adequate airway and ventilation, as well as intravenous resuscitation. The small size of the pediatric patient frequently creates difficulty in establishing adequate venous access for fluid resuscitation and this may require such initiatives as intraosseous infusion. Following the initial survey, a second, more complete examination is performed, at which time individual injuries are assessed and appropriate priorities for diagnosis and

---

Table 9-1. Priorities in Thoracic Trauma

Highest priority: Life-threatening
Tension pneumothorax
Open pneumothorax
Massive hemothorax
Flail chest
Cardiac tamponade

Second Priority: Potentially Life-threatening
Pulmonary contusion
Bronchial injuries
Myocardial contusion
Aortic rupture
Esophageal injury

Third Priority: Not Life-threatening
Simple pneumothorax
Traumatic asphyxia
Isolated diaphragmatic rupture
Chylothorax

---

treatment are determined. It is fundamental that necessary immediate therapeutic intervention are performed in conjunction with the early initial assessment of injuries (Table 9-1).

Airway Obstruction

Because of the airway's relatively small size compared to the mass of the infant or child, airway obstruction can occur easily and rapidly. If a child is noted to have airway obstruction, every attempt should be made to suction the nares and pharynx and to remove manually any foreign material. Frequently, teeth or foreign bodies from vomiting may be responsible for the obstruction, but blood and nasopharyngeal edema related to craniofacial injury can produce acute and virtually complete obstruction of the airway. If despite clearing the upper airway by suctioning there is still significant airway obstruction, an artificial airway must be inserted. Of course, either a cervical collar or inline traction of the neck must be maintained until adequate x-ray films of the cervical spine can be obtained. If endotracheal intubation is impossible, we prefer to perform rapid bronchoscopy when the patients have been able to undergo this procedure. If not, either immediate tracheostomy or cricothyrotomy is in order. Recently, we have used a rapid tracheostomy technique quite safely. Once an adequate airway has been established under these circumstances, hand ventilation has been applied and a nasogastric tube placed in the stomach to alleviate gastric distention.

Direct Injuries of the Upper Airway

External trauma to the airway in the neck is unusual, but we have encountered four patients with such injuries. All of these injuries have been related to children riding bicycles or motorcycles and being struck in the neck by outstretched cables or similar fixed structures.[8] Two of these four patients had associated cervical vertebral fractures and one also had a transected spinal cord. In both of these patients, endotracheal intubation was found to be impossible even with bronchoscopy, and immediate tracheostomy was performed below the level of the injury. In one patient, a stent was placed in the larynx, which had been fractured, and the laryngeal cartilages were reapproximated through a neck incision. In the other three patients, the injury had disconnected the trachea from the larynx, and in two, the esophagus was transected as well (Fig. 9-1) Through a broad exposure of the neck, all of these injuries were repaired following debridement, and the neck was drained. The tracheostomies have been maintained below the level of the repaired injury. It is of interest that in all four instances of significant external damage to the larynx and trachea, the skin was never lacerated. If an adequate airway has been established by tracheostomy, delayed repair of upper airway injuries may be performed in those patients with significant associated injuries and physiologic instability.[9]

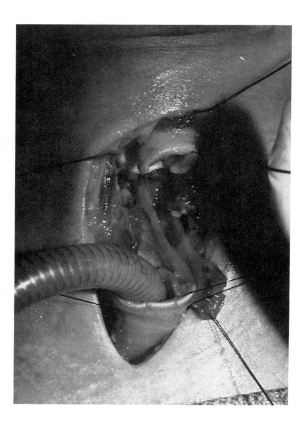

Figure 9-1. This operative photograph demonstrates complex transection of the trachea from the larynx and transection of the esophagus in a child who ran into a cable while riding a motorcycle. No laceration of the neck was present. Tracheostomy and repair by means of wide exposure in the neck was successful.

Cardiothoracic Injuries

As mentioned above, initial evaluation and treatment ordinarily must be started immediately (See Table 9-1). In patients with chest injuries, there may be simultaneous impairment of the airway, breathing mechanics, and circulation.[10,11] If a secure airway cannot be obtained by clearing obstructed airway passages and appropriate positioning of the jaw and tongue along with bag-and-mask ventilation, oral or nasotracheal intubation must be performed, taking appropriate precautions to protect the cervical spine until it can be thoroughly evaluated. We prefer to avoid tracheostomy or cricothyrotomy in patients with thoracic injuries in order to avoid unnecessary complications, and in these instances, placement of an endotracheal tube is usually possible. Once adequate intravenous lines have been established and fluid resuscitation initiated, the thorax may be evaluated both clinically and by chest x-ray.

Injuries of the Chest Wall

Mention has already been made about the pliability of the pediatric chest, which almost certainly accounts for the fact that only 40 percent of our patients with chest injuries have rib, sternal, or clavicular fractures. In most instances, it is possible to treat rib fractures with rest and analgesics, along with appropriate physical therapy measures. On the other hand, when the injuries are sufficiently extensive, there may be impairment of breathing or even paradoxical chest wall movement necessitating assisted ventilation for 10 to 14 days.[12,13] We have not always had to resort to tracheostomy under these circumstances, provided more prolonged periods of assisted ventilation have not been required. In those occasional instances in which multiple rib fractures have resulted in a flail chest, the major contribution to respiratory embarrassment has been extensive pulmonary contusion. Frequently, pneumothorax is present as well and closed tube thoracostomy drainage has been in order. In rare instances, multiple rib fractures have resulted in bleeding from intercostal arteries, occasionally this requires control by means of a thoracotomy.

Pneumothorax

The most common manifestation of thoracic injury is pneumothorax. Although simple pneumothorax may occasionally be treated by observation while the patient breathes supplemental oxygen, the opposite situation is tension pneumothorax, which may be immediately life-threatening. Consequently, pneumothorax must always be considered in the evaluation of the child with either blunt or penetrating thoracic injuries. It must be kept in mind that pneumothorax may not only result from pulmonary injury, but also from a sucking chest wound, an esophageal leak, or tracheobronchial rupture. Physical findings include diminished breath sounds on the side of the pneumothorax and shift of the trachea to the opposite side. There may be increased resonance on percussion and manifestations of subcutaneous emphysema. Although minor degrees of pneumothorax in the range of 10 percent may be treated expectantly in a patient without apparent respiratory distress by simply having the patient breathe supplemental oxygen, we have tended to use closed tube thoracostomy drainage freely in order to avoid potential sudden deterioration of the child.

In emergency situations that must be attended to before an x-ray film can be obtained, thoracentesis is an appropriate measure. A plastic-sheathed needle is best placed in the 4th or 5th intercostal space in the anterior axillary line because the chest wall is thin posterior to the pectoralis major fold.[1] The diagnosis of pneumothorax can be made in this fashion as well as that of tension pneumothorax or hemopneumothorax. The same location is appropriate for placement of an intercostal catheter and the size of the catheter should be the largest that will accommodate to the intercostal space without being compressed by the adjacent ribs. We prefer to place chest tubes directed obliquely upward through the soft tissues and the interspace, but not to tunnel tubes too far because excessive subcutaneous emphysema may accumulate. In the average child, the tube is directed posterolaterally and upward to the apex. In the infant, the tube is directed anterolaterally to the apex because in the supine position, the most superior part of the thorax is the anterior chest rather than the apex. In those instances in which there is extensive soft tissue damage and an open wound of the chest wall, the wound must be repaired sufficiently to close the thorax so that suction placed on the thoracostomy tube may re-establish negative intrathoracic pressure. Because it is the rule that pediatric patients with chest injuries have associated intra-abdominal injuries, if a child is going to be operated on for abdominal trauma, it is usually best to place a thoracostomy tube whenever there is any danger of developing a tension pneumothorax during operation.

Tension pneumothorax may cause immediate physiologic decompensation of the patient (Fig. 9-2). As mentioned above, because of the characteristic mobility of the mediastinum in children, rapid shifts may occur whenever there is progressive accumulation of air in a pleural space. Thus, angulation of the vena cavae may

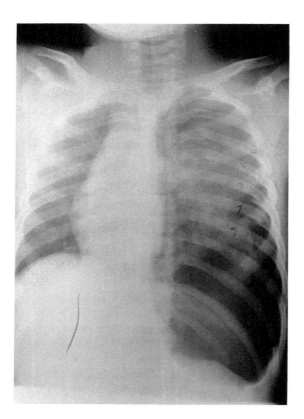

Figure 9-2. This x-ray picture demonstrates the characteristic features of tension pneumothorax, particularly wide deviation of the mediastinum. Angulation of the cavae may cause acute clinical deterioration because of impedence of venous return in the child, whose mediastinum is less fixed than that of the adult.

occur rapidly with sudden decreases in venous return and cardiac output with shock.[4] If measures are not taken immediately, death may occur.

Patients who sustain pneumothorax related to either penetrating or blunt injury should be given antibiotics because whenever lung disruption occurs, the pleural space may become contaminated. Empyema may be avoided with the use of appropriate antibiotic therapy and obliteration of pneumothorax spaces with effective tube thoracostomy drainage. Rather than simply attaching chest tubes to water seal drainage, we prefer to add suction to ensure evacuation of air and blood. In the infant, thoracostomy suction also diminishes the work of breathing; without it, the infant must increase tidal volume in order to evacuate the volume of air and fluid present within the drainage tubing circuit. Special attention must be paid to the management of assisted ventilation in those patients who have a pneumothorax related to a pulmonary leak. Generally, patients such as these have associated pulmonary contusions, and ventilator assistance is used because of poor gas exchange or associated head injuries. The minimum peak inspiratory and expiratory pressures should be used so that pulmonary leaks may seal without excessive internal pressures within the lung.[14] At times, high frequency ventilation that permits low mean airway pressures to be exerted is in order.

Hemothorax

Hemothorax virtually always occurs in association with pneumothorax, although not necessarily with tension pneumothorax. The diagnosis of hemothorax is made either with an upright chest x-ray film or by thoracentesis. Blood in the pleural space results from a vascular injury, ordinarily an intercostal artery, but may also result from a tear on the surface of the lung or from injury to major vascular structures. However, the latter is unusual, except in adolescents, because of the low incidence of penetrating injuries (Fig. 9-3). Because of the relatively low blood volume compared with body mass in small children, intrathoracic bleeding may result in shock without obvious external signs other than diminished breath sounds on the side of the injury. Generally speaking, thoracentesis to partially alleviate hemothorax is best performed in the field or in an emergency room prior to transportation. It is best to place a chest tube at the hospital where definitive therapy is to be performed because, on occasion, tube thoracostomy drainage may result in such profuse drainage of blood that it is evident that thoracotomy will be required to control the problem (Table 9-2).[15] Fortunately, tube thoracostomy drainage and restoration of normal circulating blood volume is usually all that is required for the management of most children with hemothorax. Thoracotomy will be required for hemothorax whenever there is continuing bleeding and the rate of bleeding exceeds 20 ml/kg of body weight, there is an open hemopneumothorax, evidence of aortic injury, or there has been a penetrating thoracic injury associated with massive hemorrhage.[15,16]

Occasionally, particularly in patients who have been transported long dis-

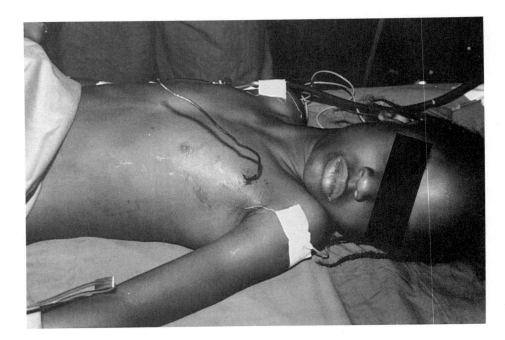

Figure 9-3. This photograph shows a child who sustained a penetrating injury of the left chest when a power lawn mower was driven over a coat hanger. This injury was associated with massive hemothorax and it was clear that the wire had traversed the chest and mediastinum. Injury to the left pulmonary artery was found and repaired.

Table 9-2. Indications for Thoracotomy in Trauma

Immediate or Shortly Following Injury
Massive pneumothorax
Cardiac tamponade
Open pneumothorax, extensive soft tissue injury
Esophageal injury
Massive air leak resulting from bronchial injury
Aortic or other vascular injury
Acute diaphragmatic rupture

Delayed
Chronic diaphragmatic rupture
Clotted hemothorax unrelieved by tube thoracostomy
Persistent chylothorax
Traumatic intracardiac defects
Evacuation of large foreign bodies
Chronic atelectasis associated with traumatic bronchial stenosis

tances, tube thoracostomy drainage does not result in sufficient evacuation of intra-thoracic clot. Inadequate evacuation of excessive amounts of blood will ordinarily lead to entrapment of lung, fibrothorax, and potentially to scoliosis, so at times thoracotomy with evacuation of clot and/or decortication should be performed.[16]

Pulmonary Contusion

Another extremely common problem related to blunt injury of the thorax in child-hood is pulmonary contusion, which may range from small areas of localized hem-orrhage to widespread bilateral pulmonary injury related to compressive forces, which may result either in blowout injuries of the lung or severe interstitial injur-ies.[14] The accumulation of hemorrhage and edema within injured areas of the lung results in an alveolar-capillary block.[17] X-ray films will reveal widespread areas of pulmonary infiltrates, hemorrhage, and fluid accumulation. There may or may not be associated pneumothorax or hemopneumothorax. In a short time, pulmonary edema occurs and there is an x-ray picture of increasing pulmonary opacification with desaturation, diminished pO_2 and increased pCO_2 characteristic of intrapul-monary shunting. Therapy is directed at maximizing the adequacy of gas exchange and preventing further deterioration and accumulation of pulmonary edema.[17] For this reason, fluid therapy is designed to promote adequate physiologic response to support vital organ function, but every effort is made to restrict the total amount of fluid administered. In critical situations, a Swann-Ganz catheter is useful as a guide to both fluid administration and ventilatory therapy by matching fluid input to pulmonary capillary wedge pressure. Diuretics are used freely; patients are para-lyzed and ventilated with just enough peak inspiratory and positive end expiratory pressure to maintain adequate oxygenation and elimination of carbon dioxide. Critically injured patients frequently develop bilateral pneumothoraces and re-quire tube thoracostomy drainage as part of their overall treatment. Severe bilat-eral pulmonary contusions are associated with a high mortality unless extreme care is used in the management of all aspects of treatment. In addition, regular bacteriologic surveillance is maintained and antibiotics are administered because infection so frequently occurs in patients with severe pulmonary contusions. We generally perform a tracheostomy in those patients who appear to require assisted or controlled ventilation for longer than 14 days.

Traumatic Asphyxia

An occasional accompaniment of pulmonary contusion is traumatic asphyxia. The typical situation involved with traumatic asphyxia is a child who has been run over by a car, under which circumstances sudden Valsalva forces are applied and pro-longed caval compression occurs.[18] Pulmonary contusions are the rule and occa-sionally pneumothorax as well, which must be treated as discussed above. Typi-cally, such children have widespread petechial hemorrhages of the face, neck and conjunctivae and they may be disoriented or even comatose, indicating that widespread capillary hemorrhage has occurred in the brain as well as the skin of the head and neck. The pulmonary problems are treated as mentioned above and appropriate treatment for head injury applied. Fortunately, permanent brain damage occurs only occasionally in patients with manifestations of traumatic asphyxia.

Bronchial Injuries

Injuries to the upper airway, including larynx and cervical trachea, have already been discussed. Injuries to the intrathoracic trachea and bronchi are unusual, but may result from either penetrating or blunt injuries. We have never encountered a tracheal injury within the chest from blunt trauma in a child, and bronchial injuries are rare, probably because of the extreme pliability and mobility of the lung and mediastinum in the pediatric age group. Typically, bronchial injury presents as pneumothorax or tension pneumothorax with some blood in the pleural space and hemoptysis. Following placement of a chest tube, massive air leak continues, a situation that should raise the suspicion that a bronchial tear may be present. Bronchoscopy may be helpful in patients who are able to tolerate this procedure, particularly if the tear is in a mainstem or intermediate bronchus. On the other hand, bronchography with Metrizamide may be a better choice for patients with critical ventilatory problems or those with tears of basilar bronchi (Fig. 9-4). Tears of the latter type may be treated with ventilatory assistance and tube thoracostomy drainage, but injuries to larger bronchi generally require direct repair through thoracotomy with ventilation of the opposite lung.[19] At times, with

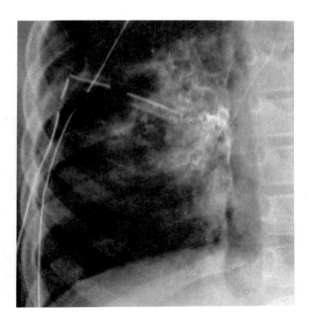

Figure 9-4. This bronchogram performed with Metrizamide demonstrates a large leak in the median basilar bronchus of the right lower lobe in a 5-year-old child who sustained severe blunt thoracic trauma in an auto accident. Severe bilateral pulmonary contusions were also present. Treatment was successful with tube thoracostomy drainage and controlled ventilation. Injuries to more proximal bronchi usually require direct repair through thoracotomy.

blunt injuries, it is preferable to repair bronchial tears early, before progressive manifestations of bilateral pulmonary contusion become evident. Occasionally, bronchial injury may result in atelectasis without there being any significant air leak. Diagnosis is made by bronchoscopy or bronchography and direct repair on a delayed basis is in order. Such repairs are usually successful. On the other hand, injury to basilar bronchi that does not seal may require lobectomy.[18]

Cardiac Injuries and Tamponade

Isolated cardiac injuries almost never occur in childhood in the absence of penetrating trauma.[20] The majority of patients who have blunt trauma have associated pulmonary contusions or other intrathoracic pathology.[4] Additionally, because the mediastinum is mobile, major cardiac and intrathoracic vascular injuries rarely occur except in the adolescent age group. Cardiac tamponade, which results either from accumulation of blood within the pericardium or air from ventilatory assistance and accumulation of interstitial air, may cause sudden cardiovascular collapse from restriction of cardiac output.[21] Such patients have diminished heart sounds, venous distention in the neck and an x-ray picture indicative of increase in the size of the cardiac silhouette. Pericardiocentesis by means of a subxiphoid approach is in order. Whenever hemopericardium resulting in cardiac tamponade is suspected, we prefer to perform pericardiocentesis in the operating room so that immediate thoracotomy can be performed if required. Drainage of the pericardial sac may be established easily through a subcostal approach to the left of the xiphoid, using a small chest tube. Pericardiocentesis is not only diagnostic, but therapeutic. Whenever thoracotomy is anticipated, standby cardiopulmonary bypass or left heart bypass should be available.

Cardiac contusion should be suspected when patients who have direct blunt injuries of the chest present with diminished cardiac output despite adequate restoration of blood volume and the diagnosis of cardiac tamponade has been eliminated.[20] MB band creatinine phosphokinase (CPK-MB) will generally be elevated in patients with myocardial contusion, and an injury pattern on EKG will be evident. Sternal fracture may be associated. Because such patients may develop sudden arrhythmias, monitoring in an intensive care unit is vital, and some patients may require inotropic augmentation of cardiac function. The majority of patients with myocardial contusions are teenagers.

Another potentially lethal injury related to the heart is aortic rupture, which is usually contained in a false aneurysm (Fig. 9-5). This problem is rare in childhood and ordinarily only occurs in the adolescent age group, which has a thorax that behaves much more like that of the adult. The majority of patients who sustain traumatic injuries to the aorta die at the scene of the injury, but occasionally such injuries are contained sufficiently to permit delayed diagnosis. Patients who demonstrate widening of the mediastinum, first rib fractures, or deviation of a nasogastric tube within the esophagus toward the right should be subjected to aortography of the aortic arch.[1] Generally, if aortic rupture is present, it occurs either at the

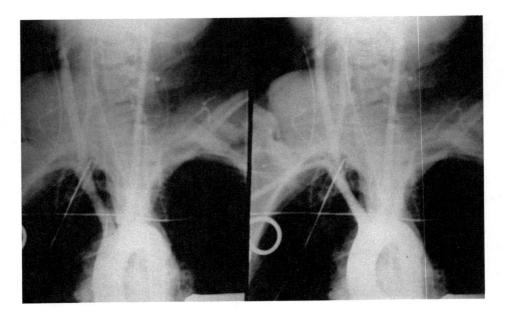

Figure 9-5. This aortogram demonstrates an intimal tear with occlusion of the right internal carotid artery and a false aneurysm of the aorta just beyond the left subclavian artery in a 17-year-old motorcycle accident victim. Such injuries are rarely encountered in younger children. Repair was performed using cardiopulmonary bypass.

takeoff of the left subclavian artery or at the site of attachment of the ligamentum arteriosum.[22] Such patients should undergo immediate repair while spinal cord and distal blood flow is maintained either through a vascular shunt or left heart bypass. Virtually all patients with aortic injuries have major associated intrathoracic and head injuries and often abdominal injuries as well. This is in contradistinction to adults, in whom isolated thoracic injuries frequently occur.[1]

On rare occasions, valvular or septal rupture may occur in association with myocardial contusions that result from severe crushing injuries to the chest.[20] Such patients will manifest progressive cardiac failure associated with new intense cardiac murmurs. Echocardiography is generally diagnostic and early repair using cardiopulmonary bypass is indicated.

Chylothorax

Chylothorax is generally manifest within a day or two following crushing injuries to the chest or penetrating injuries to the neck associated with pneumothorax. It results from disruption of the thoracic duct either at the left of the cisterna chyli or at the junction of the thoracic duct with the venous system in the neck. Chylothorax may present in either thorax. Prolonged tube thoracostomy drainage is generally effective in the treatment of patients with chylothorax, but on rare occasions, direct repair by thoracotomy may be required if excessive drainage continues longer than a month despite parenteral nutrition or the use of medium chain triglycerides in oral diets.[4] Numerous techniques have been described for the identification of the leak. We feel that it is best to perform thoracotomy on the side the chylothorax is manifested when trauma is the etiology—instead of the right thoracotomy with ligation of the cisterna chyli above the diaphragm, which has been advocated by some.

Injuries to the Diaphragm

Diaphragmatic rupture ordinarily results from blunt trauma to the upper abdomen or lower chest. Approximately 80 percent of diaphragmatic ruptures occur on the left, but occasionally right-sided and bilateral ruptures occur (Fig. 9-6).[23] Not infrequently, the diagnosis of ruptured diaphragm is not made until days to weeks later, when gradual respiratory impairment becomes evident. Chest x-ray films are diagnostic and passage of a nasogastric tube into the stomach may demonstrate the presence of the stomach within the chest on x-ray examination. A computed tomo-

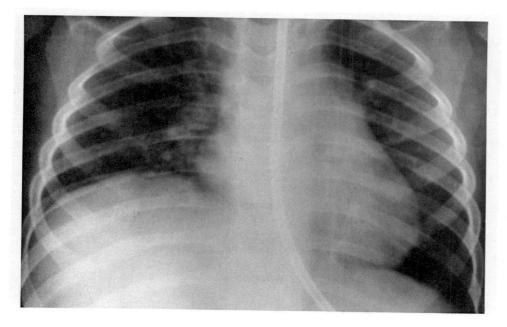

Figure 9-6. This x-ray film demonstrates right diaphragmatic rupture. Eighty percent of such ruptures occur on the left side and, when isolated, they frequently are not recognized and often do not produce symptoms for days to weeks following injury.

graphic (CT) scan with GI contrast may be diagnostic as well. We prefer to peform laparotomy for repair of diaphragmatic rupture early because of the high incidence of associated intra-abdominal injuries, particularly to the liver and spleen.[3] Characteristically, the rupture occurs in the region of the central tendon. On the other hand, patients who appears late following injury, under which circumstances associated organ injury has been eliminated and sufficient time has passed for the establishment of adhesions, repair may best be performed through thoracotomy. Any patient who has a laparotomy for acute intra-abdominal injury should have evaluation of both diaphragms as part of the abdominal exploration because injuries to the diaphragm may not be manifest immediately following injury and therefore are easily missed.

Esophageal Injuries

The most common cause of an esophageal injury in the pediatric age group is penetrating trauma, within either the thorax or the neck. Direct immediate repair is indicated under these circumstances.[24] Esophageal injuries from blunt trauma are exceedingly unusual; we have never encountered such an injury. On the other hand, blunt trauma to the cervical esophagus may result from those occasional injuries mentioned above where a child hits his or her neck on an outstretched wire while riding on a motorcycle or snowmobile. Injury to the larynx or trachea is usually associated with a shearing injury of the esophagus as well. Once again, wide exposure and direct repair is indicated with drainage and sometimes gastrostomy. The diagnosis of esophageal injury is suggested whenever mediastinal or subcutaneous emphysema is noted on either x-ray or clinical examination and no other adequate explanation, such as severe pulmonary injury, exists. The diagnosis may be confirmed by esophagram using soluble contrast material. Early repair is indicated to avoid sepsis related to mediastinitis.

References

1. Haller JA, Shermeta DW: Major thoracic trauma in children. Pediatr Clin North Am 22:341, 1975
2. Accident Facts. Chicago, National Safety Council, 1986
3. Eichelberger MR, Randolph JG: Thoracic trauma in children. Surg Clin North Am 61:1181, 1981
4. Othersen HB: Cardiothoracic injuries. In Touloukian RH (ed): Pediatric Trauma, pp 305–368. New York, John Wiley & Sons, 1978
5. O'Neill JA: Experience with iatrogenic laryngeal and tracheal stenoses. J Pediatr Surg 19:235, 1984
6. Butz RO: Length and cross section growth patterns in the human trachea. Pediatrics 42:336, 1968
7. O'Neill JA: Special pediatric emergencies. In Boswick JA (ed): Emergency Care, pp 137–147. Philadelphia, WB Saunders, 1981

8. Ashbaugh DG, Gordon JH: Traumatic avulsion of the trachea associated with cricoid fracture. J Thorac Cardiovasc Surg 69:800, 1975

9. Holinger PH, Schild JA: Pharyngeal, laryngeal and tracheal injuries in the pediatric age group. Ann Otol Rhinol Laryngol 81:538, 1972

10. Lewis FR: Thoracic trauma. Surg Clin North Am 62:97, 1982

11. Trunkey DD, Lewis FR: Chest trauma. Surg Clin North Am 60:1541, 1980

12. Cullen P: Treatment of flail chest: Use of intermittent mandatory ventilation and positive end-expiratory pressure. Arch Surg 100:1099, 1975

13. Shackford SR, Smith DE, Zarins CK et al: The management of flail chest: A comparison of ventilatory and nonventilatory treatment. Am J Surg 132:749, 1976

14. Fulton RL, Peter ET, Wilson JN: The pathophysiology and treatment of pulmonary contusions. J Trauma 10:719, 1970

15. Bodai VI, Smith P, Blaisell FW: The role of emergency thoracotomy in blunt trauma. J Trauma 22:487, 1982

16. Griffith GL, Todd EP, McMillan RD et al: Acute traumatic hemothorax. Ann Thorac Surg 26:204, 1978

17. Trinkle JK, Furman RW, Hinshaw MA et al: Pulmonary contusion, pathogenesis and effect of various resuscitative measures. Ann Thorac Surg 16:568, 1973

18. Haller JA, Danaho JS: Traumatic asphyxia in children: Pathophysiology and management. J Trauma 11:453, 1971

18. Kirsch MM, Orringer MB, Behrendt DM et al: Management of tracheobronchial disruption secondary to nonpenetrating trauma. Ann Thorac Surg 22:931, 1976

20. Golladay ES, Donaho JS, Haller JA: Special problems of cardiac injuries in infants and children. J Trauma 19:526, 1979

21. Liedtke AJ, DeMuth WE: Nonpenetrating cardiac injuries: A collective review. Am Heart J 86:687, 1973

22. Castagna J, Nelson RJ: Blunt injuries to the branches of the aortic arch. J Thorac Cardiovasc Surg 69:521, 1975

23. McCune RP, Roda CP, Eckert C: Rupture of diaphragm caused by blunt trauma. J Trauma 16:531, 1976

24. Defore WW, Mattox KL, Hanson HA et al: Surgical management of penetrating injuries of the esophagus. Am J Surg 134:734, 1987

CHAPTER 10

Liver and Spleen Trauma in Childhood

Keith T. Oldham and Michael G. Caty

T rauma is the leading cause of death and disability in children more than 1 year of age.[1,2] In the United States, approximately 15,000 childhood deaths and 2 million serious injuries related to trauma or accidental injury occur annually.[3] It is estimated that each year 19 million children, approximately 30 percent of all children in the United States, require medical care for accidental injuries.[4] The enormous magnitude of this problem has led to extensive efforts to improve trauma care at all levels. Injury prevention programs, pre-hospital care plans, and transport systems have developed rapidly in most communities during the last two decades. Initial emergency care, definitive hospital care, and rehabilitation are subjects of strong interest in virtually every large hospital. Specific causes of traumatic injuries, such as child abuse, have received a great deal of lay person and professional attention.[5]

Blunt trauma is the cause of the great majority of childhood injuries, representing approximately 80 percent of the total.[6] Penetrating injuries are less frequent and tend to be managed using algorithms that are straightforward and generally less controversial. The discussion in this chapter focuses primarily upon the evaluation and management of childhood blunt abdominal trauma that involves the liver and spleen. Penetrating injuries and adult management are reviewed briefly for purposes of comparison. Because trauma care involves an evolutionary process, some historical perspective is provided. The primary emphasis is upon practical management issues, including several specific, related controversies: blood transfusions, initial emergency evaluation, the risk of associated (hollow viscus) injury, post-splenectomy sepsis, and the continuing need for careful clinical judgement and surgical decision making.

Historical Perspective

In reports of both children and adults, the spleen is the abdominal organ most frequently injured as a result of blunt trauma.[7–9] Recently, however, several reports of computed tomography (CT) of the abdomen as a primary diagnostic maneuver have indicated that the incidence of liver injury approximates or exceeds that of the spleen.[10,11] From a practical perspective, the incidence may be considered to be roughly equal, and, as detailed below, the diagnostic and therapeutic strategies are largely the same in children. Collectively, the liver and spleen represent the large majority (approximately 75–80%) of blunt intra-abdominal injuries in children and adults. Injuries to the kidney represent approximately 15 to 10 percent of the total, and the pancreas 3 to 5 percent, although serious pancreatic ductal injury is much less common than simple contusion of the pancreas. Hollow visceral and diaphragmatic injuries are less frequent in children.[7,11,12]

Splenectomy was the unquestioned standard of therapy for traumatic splenic rupture until the 1960s and 1970s. In 1952, King and Shumaker observed that patients who had undergone splenectomy appeared to have an increased risk of death from spontaneous bacterial sepsis.[13] This was confirmed subsequently in a host of clinical reviews and laboratory investigations.[14–23] The risk of post-splenectomy sepsis is low in otherwise normal patients, including most trauma patients. It is variously estimated to be as much as 3 percent and as little as 0.5 percent or less with long-term follow-up.[15,19,22] The risk of post-splenectomy sepsis appears to be greatest in the 2 years immediately following splenectomy. Unfortunately, the mortality for post-splenectomy sepsis remains high, approximately 50 percent.[15,19,22] The pathogenesis appears to be related to the impaired ability of the splenectomized host to clear encapsulated bacteria (particularly, *Streptococcus pneumoniae*, *Haemophilus influenzae*, and *Neisseria meningitidis*) from the circulation. Important immune system defects have been described and include the following: impaired neutrophil phagocytosis; ineffective opsonization of bacteria, related in part to diminished plasma levels of complement peptide components; absent splenic clearance of neutrophils with ingested bacteria; and alterations in circulating immunoglobulin levels.[17,18,20,23–26]

In the late 1960s and 1970s, the pediatric surgical community began consistently to report successful nonoperative management of splenic injuries in children.[27–29] The enthusiasm for this approach arose from concerns related to the higher incidence of post-splenectomy sepsis in younger patients and from the frustratingly frequent experience of intraoperative observation that active bleeding from the ruptured spleen had stopped. With time, it has become clear that the reasons for this success also include the facts that the children bleed less than adults from splenic injuries, that moderate blood loss is generally well tolerated in otherwise healthy children, and that the incidence of associated abdominal hollow visceral injury is quite low in children.[11,30] The experience with adult splenic injuries is much less clear, and, it must be said, the controversy continues.[31–40] Management issues related to splenic injuries are presented in detail below.

During the 1970s, most pediatric trauma centers adopted a selective, largely nonoperative strategy for blunt splenic injuries. The evolution of imaging techniques led to widespread use of abdominal CT scanning for the initial evaluation of blunt abdominal injuries. It rapidly became clear that liver parenchymal injuries

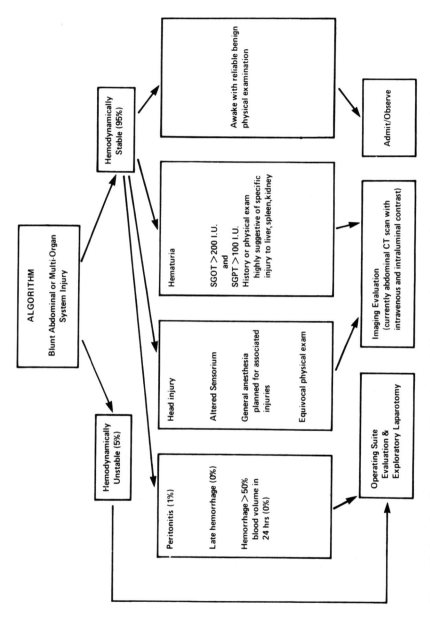

Figure 10-1. An algorithm is presented for evaluating children with blunt abdominal or multiple trauma. The percentages (%) shown reflect the findings in a recent report from Children's Hospital in Cincinnati and are reasonable approximations for most pediatric trauma centers in the United States.[11] (Reprinted with permission from Oldham KT et al: Blunt liver injury in childhood: Evolution of therapy and current perspective. Surgery 100(3): 542–549, 1986)

were present more frequently than had been suspected. It also became clear that many liver injuries could be safely managed nonoperatively. A number of studies have reported series of pediatric liver injuries with excellent results, using careful patient selection and a largely nonoperative strategy.[11,41-44] The clinical management and a summary of the existing literature is presented below.

The last two decades have seen a significant shift away from operative management of blunt liver and spleen injuries in children. The process has been more controversial in adults, and is an evolutionary rather than a revolutionary process. This chapter presents a current approach to practical clinical management issues and a review of the data that have contributed to the changes and controversies.

Splenic Injury

Splenic injury is frequent in children and must always be considered when evaluating a child with multiple trauma or with an isolated blow to the abdomen, left flank, or left chest. In an awake, stable patient who is more than 2 or 3 years of age, the physical examination is often very helpful. Localized left upper quadrant pain and tenderness without peritoneal findings are usually demonstrable. Patients with neurological abnormalities, infants and toddlers, and unstable patients are difficult to assess, and institutional diagnostic algorithms are usually employed, most often using abdominal CT scanning or diagnostic peritoneal lavage.[8,11,45,46] The approach used in our institution is illustrated in Figure 10-1.

Evaluation

The initial evaluation of the multiply injured child is presented in detail in the Specific Controversies section of this chapter. Penetrating injuries to the spleen may require laparotomy to evaluate the possibility of associated injury; this situation will not be discussed further here. Hemodynamically unstable patients with blunt abdominal trauma also require immediate laparotomy without delay for diagnostic imaging. This portion of the discussion is focused specifically upon stable patients with blunt splenic injuries. Isolated splenic injuries in children rarely result in hemodynamic instability.

When injury to a patient's spleen is possible by history, or suspected by physical examination, the diagnosis can be confirmed using one of a number of imaging techniques. It is important to note that associated injuries, such as low rib fractures on the left; contusion of the left kidney with hematuria; or pneumothorax, hemothorax, subcutaneous emphysema or pulmonary contusion secondary to lower left chest trauma, suggest splenic laceration. Ultrasound, liver and spleen radionuclide scanning, and arteriography are all useful, but provide limited information or, in the case of angiography, may be logistically unappealing and invasive.[46,47] Over a period of time, the enthusiasm for each of these techniques has diminished. Abdominal CT scanning is currently the single most useful imaging modality available for splenic and other abdominal injuries, and is therefore the most widely used.[46,48–52] Abdominal CT scanning is widely available, rapid, useful in virtually all patients, and can easily be combined with CT examination of the head or chest. Done correctly, with both intravenous and intragastric contrast, information is provided about solid viscera, retroperitoneal structures, and, to a lesser extent, the proximal gastrointestinal tract. Examples of a combined liver–spleen injury and a liver injury are shown in Figure 10-2. Obtaining and interpreting these CT scans are operator-dependent skills. Studies done by technicians without specific training and subsequently interpreted by the inexperienced are unreliable.[46,48,51] Injuries to solid viscera such as the liver and spleen may be subtle. Even with skillful assessment, injuries to the gut and pancreatic duct are very difficult to detect with CT scanning. Because these latter injuries are uncommon in children and solid visceral injuries predominate, clinical judgement by experienced surgeons will always be required to put these data into proper perspective.

Peritoneal lavage is highly sensitive for establishing the diagnosis of hemoperitoneum in both children and adults.[8] However, in children, hemoperitoneum alone or associated with a known splenic injury is not considered an absolute indication for operation. Peritoneal lavage is therefore not often helpful in decision making in this setting. In the circumstance in which serious head injury or ex-

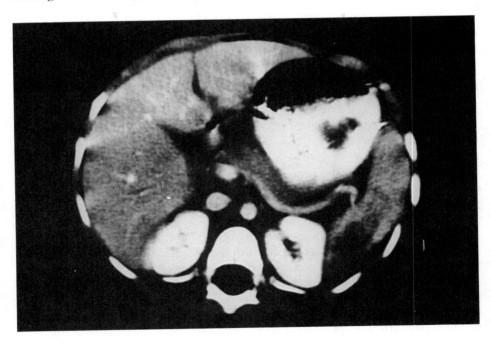

Figure 10-2. This CT scan illustrates disruption of the spleen with parenchymal hematoma, particularly posteriorly. The normal splenic vein, pancreas, and stomach are nicely shown. There is additionally a contusion to the posterior right lobe of the liver. No blood transfusion was required for this patient.

tended anesthesia for other injuries will prevent serial physical examinations, a case can be made for using diagnostic peritoneal lavage followed by laparotomy if positive. It does not seem rational to advocate diagnostic peritoneal lavage in the absence of a commitment to proceed with laparotomy if the diagnosis of hemoperitoneum is established. Most pediatric trauma centers treat the solid visceral and associated orthopedic and neurological injuries and follow the patient clinically for evidence of peritoneal inflammation, relying on the low probability of intraperitoneal hollow visceral injury in this setting. The development of peritonitis or ongoing hemorrhage requires prompt laparotomy.

Management

If the issue of associated injury is ignored, hemorrhage is the only immediate concern with regard to the injured spleen. Fortunately, bleeding from an injured spleen in a child almost always stops spontaneously and is most often stopped by the time of initial evaluation. Reports from pediatric trauma centers in Toronto,[27–29] the United States,[11,31] South Africa,[10] and Europe,[39] have shown that 70 to 95 percent of injured spleens in children can be salvaged without operation or excessive blood loss. This appears to be true regardless of the magnitude of splenic disruption demonstrated by imaging. Efforts to quantitate the degree of splenic injury for prognostic purposes by imaging have not been widely accepted.[38,53] Hemodynamic instability from an isolated splenic injury is uncommon and continuing instability after initial resuscitation is rare in children with normal spleens.

The management guidelines we have developed for isolated splenic injuries in normal children at our institution include the following:

1. Placement of appropriate intravenous catheters (usually two peripheral lines) and a nasogastric tube
2. Admission to a continuously monitored bed, usually in an intensive care unit (ICU), with frequent physical examinations and serial hematocrit determinations
3. Bed rest until splenic tenderness is resolved, usually two to four days
4. Blood transfusion only for specific clinical indications (see text below)
5. After initial resuscitation, operative exploration considered for a blood requirement greater than 50 percent of the blood volume in a 24-hour period (see text below). Hypotension or clinical evidence of continuing hemorrhage are considered relative indications for laparotomy.
6. Transfer to a ward environment when patient's condition becomes stable and no blood requirement has existed for 24 hours
7. Nasogastric tube removal and ambulation begun when splenic tenderness and ileus are resolved (usually two to four days after injury)
8. Discharge home approximately seven days after injury
9. Physical activity restriction, six to twelve weeks
10. Follow-up imaging evaluation for specific indication

It is important to point out that these are general guidelines and are not applied in any absolute fashion. There is no substitute for clinical judgement and decision making by an experienced surgical team. This issue will be discussed in detail in the portion of the chapter dealing with Specific Controversies.

Blood transfusion is required in approximately 50 percent of children with isolated splenic parenchymal injury treated nonoperatively at our institution.[54] In a large Cincinnati series of studies involving children, the incidence of blood transfusion for splenic injury treated nonoperatively was approximately 20 percent.[11] Experience in Toronto suggests that approximately one third of these children with splenic injuries require transfusion.[27] Other reports vary considerably in this regard, suggesting that the indications employed are institution-dependent. Hypotension, clinical evidence of a deficient circulating red cell mass (usually a hematocrit less than 20–25%), or expectation of significant additional blood loss from other injuries or surgical procedures are our current indications for transfusion. Maintenance of the hematocrit over 30 percent has been a general guideline in the past. However, with the current concerns regarding transfusion-related infectious diseases, a real and successful effort has been made to reduce both the amount of blood given and the number of patients who receive transfusions. It will be important therefore to distinguish between blood requirements reported historically and those in currently reported series. In asymptomatic, hemodynamically stable patients the hematocrit can be allowed to remain in the 20 to 25 percent range and the patient can be discharged on oral iron supplementation.

Splenectomy for hemorrhage after initial resuscitation and ICU admission is exceedingly uncommon using the guidelines outlined. The threshold of 50 percent of blood volume transfused in a 24-hour period after initial resuscitation for isolated splenic injuries is rarely reached. It is occasionally exceeded. This is a more difficult issue when considering combined or hepatic injuries and will be discussed further below. It is not at all clear that this nonoperative management strategy for childhood splenic injury results in either a greater incidence of transfusion or a larger volume of blood transfusion as some have suggested. On the contrary, it appears in several reports that the blood requirements may be diminished.[11,27,31]

The issues regarding operative management for splenic injury relate to the goal of obtaining control of hemorrhage while preserving as much splenic tissue as possible. Every surgeon is familiar with the experience of delivering a non-bleeding or oozing, but injured spleen into the operative field only to precipitate further bleeding. This experience is reflected in the literature by the historically high incidence of splenectomy when splenic injury is found at laparotomy for trauma.[9,32] However, a number of recent reports, including adult patients, have demonstrated successful splenic salvage in 20 to 50 percent of operated patients.[32,34,35,37] When laparotomy is required for associated injuries or in the unusual patient who presents with exsanguinating hemorrhage, the operative strategy should be to attempt to preserve the spleen. Topical hemostatic agents, splenorrhaphy or partial splenectomy may all be successfully employed.[55,56] Unfortunately, splenectomy tends to be the outcome most frequently when operation is undertaken.[9,34] Splenic artery ligation is not frequently helpful in stopping splenic hemorrhage following trauma. Arteriographic embolization for the traumatized spleen is rarely necessary or appropriate. Transplantation of the spleen or its remnants has been advocated in an effort to avoid the hazards of postsplenectomy sepsis.[57,58] However, neither clinical nor experimental studies have proven the efficacy of this approach, apparently because a normal blood supply and a residual parenchymal splenic mass of 30 to 50 percent of baseline are required for adequate function.[17,18,59]

Late hemorrhage, either in the hospital or following discharge, is distinctly uncommon in children with ruptured spleens. In a number of series, it did not occur at all.[11,27] When evaluating reports of late hemorrhage, it is important to distinguish between late recognition of hemorrhage and hemorrhage that occurs following cessation of bleeding. In the unusual circumstance in which documented late hemorrhage occurs, splenectomy should be considered. The possibility of occult splenic pathology is suggested.

It is important to recognize that the nonoperative management scheme suggested here is not appropriate for abnormal spleens. For example, deaths are reported from exsanguinating hemorrhage from ruptured spleens associated with infectious mononucleosis.[60] Other hematologic abnormalities, malignancies, or coagulopathies appear to have a similar natural history. The concurrent presence of this type of splenic pathology and splenic trauma are usually best managed by splenectomy.

This strategy appears to work well in most pediatric trauma centers. Generally in the United States this includes adolescents up to 16 to 18 years of age. In older adults, it has become clear that selected patients with splenic injuries can be managed nonoperatively. A higher incidence of associated hollow visceral injury following blunt trauma makes this approach less useful. In addition, the failure rate appears to be higher, and the tolerance of failure lower.[7,34] The key issue in adults is, of course, patient selection. It is important to carefully establish the definitions of failure (for example, the magnitude of the blood transfusion requirement), and the indications for operation in each individual report. The variability is such that it is difficult to establish a consensus among adult trauma surgeons.[31-40] This is quite different than in pediatric trauma centers, where a consensus has emerged in the last two decades. The guidelines presented here have some minor institutional variations, but are typical of most pediatric trauma centers around the world.

Liver Injury

The issue of how to properly manage blunt liver injuries is an area of significant controversy among surgeons who care for both pediatric and adult populations. Hemorrhage from liver injuries is the most common cause of death attributable to abdominal injury. In the pediatric age group, significant success has been reported by groups around the world who use a selective but largely nonoperative strategy.[11,41-44] While this appears to be a majority view among pediatric surgeons, it has not achieved the same degree of consensus that exists for splenic injuries.[61] Among adult trauma surgeons, some consider this approach heretical, and many believe a liver injury with hemoperitoneum is an absolute indication for laparotomy.[62–66] Even in children, the incidence of exsanguinating hemorrhage at initial presentation is higher (approximately 5–10%) when the liver is injured rather than the spleen.[11] Associated injuries to duodenum, pancreas or extrahepatic biliary ducts may be present. The magnitude of persistent bleeding in an ICU setting may be more, occasionally disturbingly so, than for isolated splenic injuries.

Evaluation

Like splenic injuries' association with trauma on the left side of the body, liver injuries are often associated with specific evidence of right abdominal or right chest trauma. This may be a right kidney contusion with hematuria or right-chest-wall trauma manifested by rib fractures, hemothorax, pneumothorax, or subcutaneous emphysema. The issues of the imaging evaluation are similar to those presented in this chapter's discussion regarding splenic injuries and the Specific Controversies section. Abdominal CT scanning is the procedure of choice for defining hepatic parenchymal injuries. Radionuclide scanning, ultrasound, and arteriography are useful as adjuncts, but suffer from the drawbacks previously mentioned.[67,68] In many instances, the CT scan provides a more accurate picture of the liver anatomy than can be obtained at an emergency laparotomy, where only surface anatomy is visible. Roughly 75 percent of blunt liver injuries are to the right lobe of the liver, the remainder being divided equally between those with bilobar and isolated left lobar involvement. Efforts to quantitate the degree of injury and prognosis based on volume of parenchymal disruption or relationship to portal structures have been inconsistent and unconvincing. It seems intuitive that a bilobar "explosion" type of injury with fragmentation of parenchyma should be more serious than a simple laceration. Indeed, this appears to be the case, but it has proven difficult to quantitate. For the evaluation of liver injuries, the cautionary notes regarding careful, meticulous attention to the technical aspects of CT scanning are critical.[51] The accuracy described in this and other reviews can only be obtained under optimal conditions. Less than this will only yield confusing or misleading data.

Decisions regarding initial evaluation for liver injury depend upon the management preferences of the senior trauma surgeon. Hemodynamically unstable patients do not require discussion. All would agree that emergency laparotomy is mandatory. If the source of bleeding is unclear, diagnostic peritoneal lavage will readily confirm the diagnosis of hemoperitoneum. Penetrating injuries to the liver are also not a point of dispute; laparotomy without delay is required. The initial evaluation becomes controversial in the hemodynamically stable patient with suspected liver injury and no compelling reason for laparotomy, such as an obvious associated hollow visceral injury. In adults, both peritoneal lavage and CT scanning are commonly done;[51] the former is favored by those who consider hemoperitoneum an indication for laparotomy. Even among advocates, CT scans are done in a minority of cases of adult liver injury. Trunkey and associates report using CT in only 14 percent of 2000 adult patients with abdominal trauma.[51] For children, most trauma surgeons prefer an imaging evaluation. Because abdominal CT scanning provides a great deal more information about the liver, spleen, kidneys, and other retroperitoneal structures on a single examination, this is the preference over ultrasound, radionuclide scanning, or arteriography.

Indications for CT scanning include those outlined in the management algorithm proposed in Figure 10-1. It is important to note that emergency room determinations of serum transaminase levels are useful for selecting patients to undergo CT scanning. A corollary finding in a review of the Cincinnati pediatric experience with CT scans and liver trauma was that transaminase enzyme elevations in serum were a consistent finding immediately after hepatic trauma.[69] SGOT and SGPT levels greater than 200 IU and 100 IU, respectively, were found for all children with liver injuries. Below this threshold no injuries occurred and above this threshold the probability of liver injury exceeded 60 percent. These threshold values are useful for emergency room screening, and when exceeded are considered in our institution to be an indication to obtain an abdominal CT scan.

Management

Approximately 5 to 10 percent of children with blunt liver injuries present with exsanguinating hemorrhage in the emergency room. This is not a subtle diagnosis. Refractory hypotension and shock are obvious and immediate laparotomy without diagnostic delay is required. These children usually have major vascular injuries, usually hepatic vein or retrohepatic vena cava lacerations associated with large parenchymal disruptions. Operative management is likely to require major resectional debridement or lobectomy to control the hemorrhage.

However, the majority of children with liver injuries are hemodynamically stable when first evaluated in the emergency room. The imaging evaluation is discussed above and the management guidelines are generally similar to those provided for splenic injuries. The magnitude of the transfusion requirement tends to be higher for liver injuries. In the largest reported series, only 20 percent of children with blunt liver injuries required transfusion.[11] In our institution, the incidence of blood transfusion is approximately 30 percent.[70] The ileus and right upper quadrant pain may be more persistent and the ICU stay longer than for isolated splenic injuries.

A small number of children have persistent bleeding with an ongoing blood requirement. These patients tend to have more complex bursting injuries, which may be bilobar. The threshold of 50 percent of blood volume replacement in 24 hours is not often reached, but it may be exceeded in a hemodynamically stable patient. Early operative management may precipitate exsanguinating hemorrhage, requiring a major hepatic resection with its attendant high mortality. It appears that certain patients with these complex, life-threatening injuries can be stabilized in an ICU setting with transfusion and avoid emergency surgical procedures, which carry operative mortality rates as high as 10 to 50 percent.[62-64] Late complications may occur in 10 to 15 percent of these patients.[11] These take the form of bile peritonitis, which may require delayed laparotomy for debridement and drainage; at these later times, the problem of acute hemorrhage appears to be substantially diminished. Current techniques of percutaneous CT or ultrasound-directed catheter drainage may obviate the need for some of these open procedures. Hemobilia is reported, but is preferentially managed by angiographic embolization, which is ordinarily quite safe. Disruption of the extrahepatic biliary tract may occur from blunt trauma and the diagnosis may well be delayed because CT scanning is unlikely to detect this problem (Figure 10-3); however, elective late reconstruction is likely to be at least as successful as immediate reconstruction in the face of active hemorrhage. Success with this selective but primarily nonoperative strategy results in survival in up to 96 percent of all children with injured livers.[11] Table 10-1

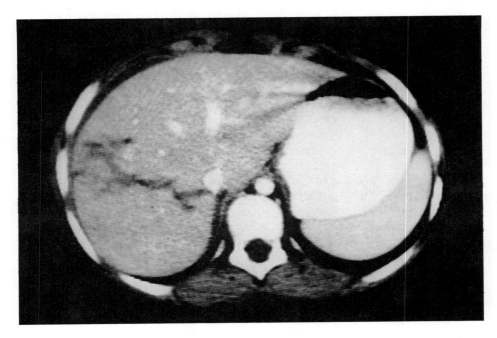

Figure 10-3. This CT scan demonstrates a deep parenchymal fracture in the right lobe of the liver extending tranversely to the inferior vena cava. This anatomy would be very difficult to discern at laparotomy. This patient was successfully managed nonoperatively without blood transfusion. She presented with hemobilia 16 days after injury and this was successfully managed angiographically.

Table 10-1. Pediatric Liver Trauma

Author	Total Number	Nonoperated	Nonoperated and Alive	Nonoperated and Complication	Operated	Operated and Alive
Karp (1983)	17	15	15	0	2 (1 late)	2
Cywes (1983)	23	19	19	1	4 (1 late)	4
Giacomantonio (1984)	32	14	14	0	18	11
Grisoni (1984)	12	9	8	0	3	0
Oldham (1986)	53	47	47	2	6 (2 late)	4
Totals	137	104 (76%)	103 (99%)	3 (3%)	33 (24%)	21 (64%)

Five large series of pediatric liver trauma from around the world in the 1980s are summarized. [11, 41–44] Seventy six percent of the selected patients in these series were successfully managed without operation and 91 percent of all patients survived. Ninety nine percent of the unoperated patients survived. These results demonstrate that a selective, but largely nonoperative management strategy can be safely used in children (see text for discussion).

provides a summary of several of the largest experiences with unoperated liver injuries in children.[11,12,41,43,44] These compare quite favorably with most reports emphasizing prompt laparotomy. These latter reports continue to have mortality rates of 10 to 30 percent.[62–66] In addition, most operative series have similar incidences (10–15%) of such complications as late hemorrhage, bile peritonitis, or hemobilia.

The requirements for the approach advocated here for children with liver injuries include an experienced ICU team familiar with the care of surgical and trauma patients; a group of surgeons and surgical house officers committed to full-time care of trauma patients as the primary and responsible physicians; and full support and immediate availability of all hospital facilities, operating rooms, anesthesia staff, and blood bank facilities. If these conditions are not fulfilled, routine laparotomy may be a safer approach. Given these commitments, selective but largely nonoperative management of blunt liver injuries is a safe and reasonable alternative in children.[71]

In adults, the data are not necessarily convincing for this approach. However, a number of authors have reported successful nonoperative management in small numbers of carefully selected adult patients with liver injuries.[31,51,72,73] The cautionary comments in the previous discussion of adult splenic trauma are relevant to the liver as well.

Specific Controversies
Initial Evaluation for Childhood Trauma

A number of approaches to the initial evaluation of the injured child have been described. These may be quite complex.[45] Two key elements for success in designing an institutional approach are prospective planning and education of the entire trauma team, and simplicity. Routines are often the safest approach in a system that includes many different specialty groups with individuals at different levels of training. The routines must remain subject to individualized judgements by senior surgeons. Our institutional guidelines are illustrated in Figure 10-1.[11] These are purposely simple, but reflect in general terms an approach used in pediatric trauma centers around the world. The percentages shown in Figure 10-1 reflect the approximate frequencies of these specific problems. The large majority (95%) of children with blunt abdominal or multi-system injury undergo initial evaluation by abdominal CT scanning. In most cases, this is definitive and represents the single diagnostic test done. Most authors report some intra-abdominal pathology on 20 to 50 percent of CT scans obtained. Clearly this yield depends upon the indications employed. Note that diagnostic peritoneal lavage is not routinely used in treatment of children. Peritoneal lavage is highly sensitive for demonstrating hemoperitoneum (95–98% accuracy).[8] Its drawbacks include a lack of sensitivity for retroperitoneal injury and ruptured diaphragm, and a high incidence of false positive lavage with pelvic fractures.[8,51] In addition, patients with previous surgery are not good candidates, and, most importantly, laparotomy done solely for hemoperitoneum has a high probability of being nontherapeutic. In children, the usefulness of diagnostic peritoneal lavage is usually limited to the neurologically impaired, as described in the discussion of evaluation for splenic trauma.

Operative Management of the Injured Liver

The proper operative management for the injured liver remains contentious because it requires difficult intraoperative decision making. Fortunately, this set of issues is confronted infrequently in pediatric trauma patients today. When laparotomy is performed for hemoperitoneum or to explore an associated intra-abdominal injury, the liver is generally not bleeding significantly despite parenchymal injury. In this circumstance nothing need be done. External drainage, topical hemostatic agents, and simple suture repair may be performed, but these maneuvers are often unnecessary. For larger injuries, large mattress suture hepatorraphy, suture ligature of specific bleeding points, omental packing, use of the Pringle maneuver (temporary occlusion of the hepatoduodenal ligament), hepatic artery ligation, or resectional debridement may be necessary. Recent literature argues strongly for surgical restraint in handling these complex injuries.[74–77] The successful use of nonoperative management in children argues against aggressive debridement of nonbleeding, but marginally viable liver parenchyma. More complex injuries may require formal hepatic lobectomy. Transplantation is reported for otherwise unreconstructable injuries. Injuries to the hepatic veins or retrohepatic vena cava (IVC) may require median sternotomy with insertion of an atrial-caval shunt. However, the blood loss is still very high, and mortality is at least 50 to 90 percent with this approach.[62,78] This maneuver is a matter of personal preference for the surgeon, but the enthusiasm of a decade ago is currently diminished. Simple occlusion of the infrahepatic and suprahepatic IVC is probably equally effective. Hemostasis can usually be provided by packing. This is generally a temporary maneuver, but may allow transfer of a patient to another institution or allow the completion of resuscitation prior to definitive surgical therapy. Resuscitation in this circumstance may very well include correction of hypothermia and a coagulopathy. In the last five years, enthusiasm for this technique has undergone a resurgence.[79] This is clearly a technique to be added to the inventory of alternatives available to deal with complex liver injuries, although it is not suitable for major venous injuries. A detailed discussion of operative techniques is beyond the scope of this chapter, but several recent reviews are available.[74–77,80]

Associated Injuries

Fortunately, the incidence of hollow visceral injuries in children following blunt trauma is low. In virtually all series of multiply injured children or children with isolated blunt abdominal trauma, the incidence is less than 5 percent, usually to 1 to 2 percent.[10,11] One recent exception is a report from South Africa with an 18 percent incidence of intestinal injury in a study group of over 50 children.[81] This unusually high incidence probably reflects referral patterns to a tertiary-care children's hospital and perhaps some environmental differences with regard to the mechanisms of injury. It is at substantial variance with most reports.[10,11] The usual low incidence of these injuries in children represents a significant difference from the adult population, in which this incidence may be 10 to 15 percent.[7,82] This allows the pediatric surgeon to accept a more conservative approach toward exploratory surgery to rule out perforation of a hollow visceral organ. Bowel injuries are detectable on serial physical examination and are repairable without increased mortality.[83] The same appears to be true for rupture of the diaphragm. Renal injuries are relatively common in children, but, even more than for liver and spleen trauma, a consensus exists that nonoperative management is desirable. Except for instances of renal pedicle vascular injury, renal parenchyma is inevitably better preserved when operation is delayed or avoided altogether. This can usually be achieved because the retroperitoneal location of the kidneys makes tamponade of bleeding highly probable.

Pancreatic injuries are troublesome to diagnose regardless of approach. Most pancreatic injuries in children with blunt trauma are contusions that can be demonstrated on CT scan and confirmed by clinical exam and serum amylase and lipase determinations. Major pancreatic ductal injuries, usually fractures over the vertebral column, may be combined with duodenal injury and detected at laparotomy. Neither CT scan nor peritoneal lavage is sensitive for this injury. Clinical judgment will remain a necessity.

Head injuries and orthopedic injuries are frequent in children with blunt trauma and the overall morbidity and mortality are directly related to the severity of these associated problems. Aggressive multidisciplinary care in a trauma center is essential for an optimal outcome.

Pneumococcal Vaccination and Post-splenectomy Penicillin Prophylaxis

The risk of bacterial sepsis in asplenic patients, particularly young children, is well documented.[13,22] As was noted in the Historical Perspective section of this chapter, the incidence is generally thought to be less than 1 percent following splenectomy for trauma.[16,22] In 1978, polyvalent pneumococcal vaccine became commercially available and is currently recommended for children and adults who have had or will undergo splenectomy. Theoretically, this provides protection against some strains of pneumococcal organisms, the most common cause of post-splenectomy sepsis. Because not all pneumococcal organisms are covered, and because other organisms such as *Neisseria meningitidis* or *Haemophilus influenzae* may be the cause, this can be regarded as a partial solution at best.[23,84] The suggestion has been made that the incidence of post-splenectomy sepsis is diminished in recent years, but continued vigilance will be necessary.

In addition, lifelong oral penicillin prophylaxis is advocated by some, perhaps most, surgeons following splenectomy. Patient compliance is a concern with this approach. This strategy is theoretically appealing and appears to be benign in character.[23,85] To date there is no convincing data establishing efficacy; indeed, failure has been reported. Confirmation of validity for this approach awaits long-term prospective studies.

Splenic autotransplantation has also been proposed to ameliorate the problem of post-splenectomy sepsis. Although some experimental animal and human data would support this concept, this has yet to be proven reliable in clinical human use.[23,57,58] Definitive support for this approach has not developed, in children largely because few splenectomies are currently performed following trauma. The best solution to the problem of post-splenectomy sepsis is preservation of the spleen whenever possible.[23]

Blood Transfusions

The hazards of blood transfusion have been emphasized in the last decade by the appearance of the acquired immunodeficiency syndrome (AIDS) virus in the blood supply. While the risk of AIDS transmission is low with current ELISA screening (estimated incidence, 1 per 100,000 units), it remains a serious and emotionally charged problem.[86] Hepatitis transmission by means of transfused blood is a much larger issue in terms of frequency. It is estimated that the frequency of post-transfusion hepatitis is 6 to 10 percent in most donor pools and is most frequently non-A non-B hepatitis.[83] Of the affected patients, 20 to 50 percent may develop chronic hepatitis. Luna and Dellinger have estimated the probability of death secondary to a 4-unit blood transfusion to be 0.56 percent.[16] Because of these concerns, some have questioned the wisdom of nonoperative therapy for liver and spleen trauma. This criticism assumes that the transfusion requirement is greater when nonoperative management is selected for liver and spleen trauma. This assumption is unproven. Our data and that of others suggest that this may not be true.[11,27,31] In one large series, only 20 percent of children with spleen and liver injuries received a transfusion.[11] In a current review at our institution, 30 percent of children with injured livers and 50 percent of those with splenic injuries received transfusions.[31] Splenic injuries and most liver injuries do not usually bleed further after initial emergency presentation.

In addition, complex and bilobar liver injuries may very well require larger blood transfusion volumes or prove to be unsalvageable if surgical exploration is undertaken. We have cared for several hemodynamically stable children with liver injuries who were transferred to our institution for complex problems related to operations and massive blood loss associated with surgical procedures.

Given the hazards of transfusion-related viral diseases, it is prudent to provide blood transfusion only when required for the treatment of a specific problem. It is not necessary to maintain the hematocrit at some arbitrary level in a healthy, asymptomatic child. For this reason, the frequency and volume of blood transfusions at our own institution have diminished.

Clinical Judgment

The guidelines presented in this chapter are necessarily general. Variations from the routine are the rule in traumatized children. Individualized judgments by surgeons experienced in the care of pediatric trauma patients will always be necessary. Although most pediatric trauma patients do not require operations for their liver or spleen injuries, their management requires appropriate and continuously available support from the ICU, operating rooms, anesthesia staff, blood bank, and hospital. The consequences of failing to recognize problems when they arise, or being unprepared to act immediately, are potentially life-threatening for the patient. The role of a senior surgeon in the decision-making process for these children is essential and cannot be delegated to junior house officers, pediatricians, intensivists or others. Given these cautions, children have proven quite resilient. In the absence of serious head injury, children who arrive alive at a hospital can be expected to survive in almost every instance.

Conclusion

The management of children with blunt abdominal or multiple trauma resulting in injury to the spleen or liver has been reviewed. Emphasis is placed upon the evolution of nonoperative management for selected patients. Most children can be successfully managed in this fashion. A number of cautions are presented and the continuing need for careful clinical judgement by surgeons experienced in the care of trauma patients is emphasized.

References

1. Haller JA: Problems in children's trauma. J Trauma 10:269–271, 1970
2. Harris BH, Eichelberger M, Haller JA, O'Neill JA: Trauma in children. Contemp Surg 22:123–129, 1983
3. Gratz RR: Accidental injury in childhood: A literature review on pediatric trauma. J Trauma 19(8):551–555, 1979
4. White House Conference on Children: Profiles on Children. Washington DC, 1970
5. Kempe CH, Silverman FN, Steele BF et al: The battered child syndrome. JAMA 181:17–24, 1962
6. Committee on Trauma: Advanced Trauma Life Support Instructor Manual. Chicago, American College of Surgeons, 1984
7. Cox EF: Blunt abdominal trauma: A 5-year analysis of 870 patients requiring celiotomy. Ann Surg 199(4):467–474, 1984
8. Drew R, Perry JF, Fischer RP: The experience of peritoneal lavage for blunt trauma in children. Surg Gynecol Obstet 145:885–888, 1977
9. Mustard RA, Hanna SS, Blair G et al: Blunt splenic trauma: Diagnosis and management. Can J Surg 27:330–333, 1984
10. Cywes S, Kibel SM, Bass DH: Pediatric trauma in South Africa. In Coran AG, Harris BH (eds): Pediatric Trauma: Proceedings of the Third National Conference, pp 205–221. Philadelphia, JB Lippincott, 1990

11. Oldham KT, Guice KS, Ryckman F et al: Blunt liver injury in childhood: Evolution of therapy and current perspective. Surgery 100(3):542–549, 1986
12. Kearney PA, Vahey T, Burney RE, Glazer G: Computed tomography and diagnostic peritoneal lavage in blunt abdominal trauma: Their combined role. Arch Surg 124:344–347, 1989
13. King H, Shumacker HB: Splenic studies: Susceptibility to infection after splenectomy performed in infancy. Ann Surg 136(2):239–242, 1952
14. Dickerman JD: Bacterial infection and the asplenic host: A review. J Trauma 16(8):662–668, 1976
15. Eraklis AJ, Filler RM: Splenectomy in childhood: A review of 1413 cases. J Pediatr Surg 7(4):382–388, 1972
16. Luna GK, Dellinger P: Nonoperative observation therapy for splenic injuries: A safe therapeutic option? Am J Surg 153:462–468, 1987
17. Malangoni MA, Dawes LG, Droege EA, Almagro UA: The influence of splenic weight and function on survival after experimental pneumococcal infection. Ann Surg 202(3):323–328, 1985
18. Malangoni MA, Dawes LG, Droege EA et al: Splenic phagocytic function after partial splenectomy and splenic autotransplantation. Arch Surg 120:275–278, 1985
19. O'Neil BJ and McDonald JC: The risk of sepsis in the asplenic adult. Ann Surg 194(6):775–778, 1981
20. Pearson HA, Spencer RP, Cornelius EA: Functional asplenia in sickle-cell anemia. N Engl J Med 281:923–926, 1969
21. Scher KS, Scott-Conner C, Jones CW, Wroczynski AF: Methods of splenic preservation and their effect on clearance of pneumococcal bacteremia. Ann Surg 202(5):595–599, 1985
22. Singer DB: Postsplenectomy sepsis. In Rosenberg HS, Bolande RP (eds): Perspectives in Pediatric Pathology, vol 1, pp 285–311. Chicago, Year Book Medical Publishers, 1973
23. Traub A, Giebink GS, Smith C et al: Splenic reticuloendothelial function after splenectomy, spleen repair, and spleen autotransplantation. N Engl J Med 317(25):1559–1564, 1987
24. Bjornson AB, Lobel JS: Direct evidence that decreased serum opsonization of *Streptococcus pneumoniae* via the alternative complement pathway in sickle cell disease is related to antibody deficiency. J Clin Invest 79:388–398, 1987
25. Linne T, Eriksson M, Lannergren K et al: Splenic function after nonsurgical management of splenic rupture. J Ped 105(2):263–265, 1984
26. Phillippart AI, Hight DW: Splenectomy in childhood: Altered concepts of management. Am J Ped Hematol Oncol 2(1):61–68, 1980
27. Filler RM: Experience with the management of splenic injuries. Aust NZ J Surg 54:443–445, 1984
28. Upadhyaya P, Simpson JS: Splenic trauma in children. Surg Gynecol Obstet 126:781–790, 1968
29. Wesson DE, Filler RM, Ein SH et al: Ruptured spleen: When to operate? J Ped Surg 16(3):324–326, 1981
30. Wesson DE: Abdominal injuries in children. Can J Surg 27(5): 472–474, 1984
31. Delius RE, Frankel W, Coran AG: A comparison between operative and nonoperative management of adult and pediatric patients with blunt injuries to the liver and spleen. Surgery (in press)

32. Flancbaum L, Dauterive A, Cox EF: Splenic conservation after multiple trauma in adults. Surg Gynecol Obstet 162:469–473, 1986

33. Hunter RA, Kiroff GK, Jamieson GG: The injured spleen: Should consideration be given to conservative management? Aust NZ J Surg 54:129–135, 1984

34. Malangoni MA, Levine AW, Droege EA et al: Management of injury to the spleen in adults. Ann Surg 200(6):702–705, 1984

35. Moore FA, Moore EE, Moore GE, Millikan JS: Risk of splenic salvage after trauma: Analysis of 200 adults. Am J Surg 148:800–805, 1984

36. Moss JF, Hopkins WM: Nonoperative management of blunt splenic trauma in the adult: A community hospital's experience. J Trauma 27(3):315–318, 1987

37. Nallathambi MN, Ivatury RR, Wapnir I et al: Nonoperative management versus early operation for blunt splenic trauma in adults. Surg Gynecol Obstet 166:252–258, 1988

38. Resciniti A, Fink MP, Raptopoulos V et al: Nonoperative treatment of adult splenic trauma: Development of a computer tomographic scoring system that detects appropriate candidates for expectant management. J Trauma 128(6):828–831, 1988

39. Solheim K, Hoivik B: Changing trends in the diagnosis and management of rupture of the spleen. Injury 16(4):221–226, 1985

40. Zucker K, Browns K, Rossman D et al: Nonoperative management of splenic trauma. Arch Surg 119: 400–403, 1984

41. Cywes S, Rode H, Millar AJW: Blunt liver trauma in children: Nonoperative management. J Pediatr Surg 20:14–18, 1985

42. Giacomantonio M, Filler RM, Rich RH: Blunt hepatic trauma in children: Experience with operative and nonoperative management. J Pediatr Surg 19:519–522, 1984

43. Grisoni ER, Gauderer ML, Ferron J, Izant RJ: Nonoperative management of liver injuries following blunt abdominal trauma in children. J Pediatr Surg 19:515–518, 1984

44. Karp MP, Cooney DR, Pros GA et al: The nonoperative management of pediatric hepatic trauma. J Pediatr Surg 18:512–518, 1983

45. Eichelberger MR and Randolph JG: Pediatric trauma: An algorithm for diagnosis and therapy. J Trauma 23(2):91–97, 1983

46. Karp MP, Cooney DR, Berger PE et al: The role of computed tomography in the evaluation of blunt abdominal trauma in children. J Pediatr Surg 16(3):316–323, 1981

47. Froelich JW, Simeone JF, McKusick KA et al: Radionuclide imaging and ultrasound in liver/spleen trauma: A prospective comparison. Radiol 145:457–461, 1982

48. Federle MP: Abdominal trauma: The role and impact of computed tomography. Invest Radiol 16(4):260–268, 1981

49. Federle MP, Crass RA, Jeffrey RB, Trunkey DD: Computed tomography in blunt abdominal trauma. Arch Surg 117:645–650, 1982

50. Jeffrey RB, Laing FC, Federle MP, Goodman PC: Computed tomography of splenic trauma. Radiology 41(3):729–732, 1981

51. Meredith JW, Trunkey DD: CT scanning in acute abdominal injuries. Surg Clin North Am 68(2):255–268, 1988

52. Toombs BD, Lester RG, Ben-Menachem Y, Sandler CM: Computed tomography in blunt trauma. Radiol Clin North Am 19(1):17–35, 1981

53. Buntain WL, Gould HR, Maull KI: Predictability of splenic salvage by computed tomography. J Trauma 28(1):24–34, 1988

54. Oldham KT, Caty MG: Unpublished data

55. Burrington JD: Surgical repair of a ruptured spleen in children. Arch Surg 112:417–419, 1977

56. Ratner MH, Garrow E, Valda V et al: Surgical repair of the injured spleen. J Pediatr Surg 12(6):1019–1025, 1977
57. Pabst R, Kamran D: Autotransplantation of splenic tissue. J Pediatr Surg 21(2):120–124, 1986
58. Patel J, Williams JS, Shmigel B, Hinshaw JR: Preservation of splenic function by autotransplantation of traumatized spleen in man. Surgery 39:683–689, 1981
59. Moore GE, Stevens RE, Moore EE, Aragon GE: Failure of splenic implants to protect against fatal postsplenectomy infection. Am J Surg 146(3):413–414, 1983
60. Jones TJ, Pugsley WG, Grace RH: Fatal spontaneous rupture of the spleen in asymptomatic infectious mononucleosis. J R Coll Surg Edinb 30(6):398, 1985
61. Bass BL, Eichelberger MR, Schisgall R, Randolph JG: Hazards of nonoperative therapy of hepatic injury in children. J Trauma 24(11):978–982, 1984
62. Cogbill TH, Moore EE, Jurkovich GJ et al: Severe hepatic trauma: A multi-center experience with 1,335 liver injuries. J Trauma 28(10):1433–1438, 1988
63. Defore WW, Mattox KL, Jordan GL, Beall AC: Management of 1,590 consecutive cases of liver trauma. Arch Surg 111:493–497, 1976
64. Douglas RG, Holdaway CM, Shaw JH: Hepatic trauma in Auckland. Aust NZ J Surg 58(4):307–14, 1988
65. Feliciano DV, Mattox KL, Jordan GL et al: Management of 1,000 consecutive cases of hepatic trauma (1979–1984). Ann Surg 204(4):438–445, 1986
66. Trunkey DD, Shires GT, McClelland R: Management of liver trauma in 811 consecutive patients. Ann Surg 179(5):722–727, 1974
67. Sclafani SJA, Shaftan GW, McAuley J et al: Interventional radiology in the management of hepatic trauma. J Trauma 24(3):256–262, 1984
68. Weissmann HS, Byun KJC, Freeman LM: Role of Tc-99m IDA scintigraphy in the evaluation of hepatobiliary trauma. Semin Nucl Med 8(3):199–222, 1983
69. Oldham KT, Guice, KS, Kaufman RA et al: Blunt hepatic injury and elevated hepatic enzymes: A clinical correlation in children. J Pediatr Surg 19(4)457–461, 1984
70. Oldham KT, Caty MG: Unpublished data
71. Oldham KT, Guice KS: Letter to the Editor: Blunt hepatic injury in children. Surgery 103:717–718, 1988
72. Athey GN, Rahman SU: Hepatic haematoma following blunt injury: Non-operative management. Injury 13(4):302–306,
73. Farnell MB, Spencer MP, Thompson E et al: Nonoperative management of blunt hepatic trauma in adults. Surgery 104(4):748–756, 1988
74. Moore FA, Moore EE, Seagraves A: Nonresectional management of major hepatic trauma: An evolving concept. Am J Surg 150(6):725–729, 1985
75. Pretre R, Mentha G, Huber O et al: Hepatic trauma: Risk factors influencing outcome. Br J Surg 75(6):520–524, 1988
76. Stain SC, Yellin AE, Donovan AJ: Hepatic trauma. Arch Surg 123(10):1251–1255, 1988
77. Witte CL, Zukoski CF: A rational approach to serious blunt hepatic injury. Am Surg 49(8):446–453, 1983
78. Rovito PF: Atrial caval shunting in blunt hepatic vascular injury. Ann Surg 205(3):318–321, 1987
79. Baracco-Gandolfo V, Vidarte O, Baracco-Miller V, DelCastillo M: Prolonged closed liver packing in severe hepatic trauma: Experience with 36 patients. J Trauma 26(8):754–756, 1986
80. Lucas CE, Ledgerwood AM: Prospective evaluation of hemostatic techniques for liver injuries. J Trauma 16(6):442–451, 1976

81. Kovacs GZ, Davies MRQ, Saunders W et al: Hollow viscus rupture due to blunt trauma. Surg Gynecol Obstet 163:552–554, 1986
82. Dauterive AH, Flancbaum L, Cox EF: Blunt intestinal trauma: A modern-day review. Ann Surg 201(2):198–203, 1985
83. Debeugny P, Canarelli L, Bonevalle M et al: Intestinal perforation in abdominal contusions in children. Chir Pediatr 29(1):7–10, 1988
84. Applebaum PC, Shaikh BS, Widome MD et al: Fatal pneumococcal bacteremia in a vaccinated, splenectomized child. N Engl J Med 300:203–204, 1979
85. Powell RW, Blaylock WE, Hoff CJ, Chartrand SA: The efficacy of postsplenectomy sepsis prophylactic measures: The role of penicillin. J Trauma 28(6):1285–1288, 1988
86. Rubin RH, Tolkoff-Rubin NE: Post transfusion viral infections. Transplant Proc 20(6):1112–1117, 1988

CHAPTER 11

Bowel Injuries

Julie A. Long and Arvin I. Philippart

*I*n contrast to adults, pediatric trauma is characterized by a greater incidence and significance of head injury; a higher ratio of blunt to penetrating trauma, particularly before adolescence; and a larger number of injuries that can be managed successfully without operation. Additionally, intestinal injury is less frequently seen in children than in adults. The radiologic evaluation of intestinal trauma has not shown the same improvement over the past decade as has evaluation of solid visceral injury. Thus, there remains a major emphasis on clinical acumen, which requires knowledge of mechanisms and patterns of injury. Currently available diagnostic techniques complement, but do not replace the need for frequent and repetitive clinical assessments.

The National Institute on Disability and Rehabilitation Research Pediatric Trauma Registry (PTR) currently reports that 7.3 percent of more than 10,000 children hospitalized for trauma had thoracoabdominal injuries. A recent 5-year review of our experience at the Children's Hospital of Michigan (CHM) revealed 262 admissions for suspected abdominal trauma, representing 7.1 percent of all trauma admissions. Of this group, 19 percent underwent laparotomy.

It has been well established that patterns of injury differ between children and adults. In a recent review of 6301 adults and 1275 children with blunt abdominal trauma, Fischer and associates found a significantly higher incidence of gastrointestinal disruption in adults than in children.[1] The major differences between pediatric and adult abdominal trauma can be explained by the smaller size and structure of the pediatric patient and differences in the mechanisms of injury. Because on a child the force of blunt impact is distributed over a larger proportion of the body, multiple injury is more common; head and extremity injuries are particularly frequent. Falls and bicycle injuries are much more common causes of injury in children. The PTR reports an 84 percent incidence of blunt trauma and a 12 percent incidence of penetrating trauma. In urban centers, the incidence of penetrating trauma is higher, for example, a 20 percent incidence of penetrating trauma has been reported at the CHM.

Much as children's surgeons have held the responsibility of expanding trauma knowledge to include those differences found in pediatric trauma, it is imperative for children's surgeons to remain informed of practice in adult trauma surgery and when appropriate to apply that knowledge to the care of children. Examples of changing practice are the emergence of computed tomographic (CT) scanning and diagnostic peritoneal lavage over the past 20 years, in contrast to the earlier complete reliance on physical examination. The field's more extensive experience with adult trauma is also relevant to the epidemiologic shift to increasing trauma volume and incidence of penetrating injury in children. Current emphasis is on not only patient salvage and rehabilitation, but also increased diagnostic accuracy (with an eye to the risks and costs of less than accurate patient selection for operative intervention).

Shaftan's landmark 1960 paper showed that not all patients with presumed abdominal trauma require laparotomy.[2] To decrease the human error in assessing abdominal tenderness, numerous ancillary tests have been advocated to evaluate intra-abdominal injury. Only abdominal CT scan and diagnostic peritoneal lavage (DPL) are considered currently to have routine applicability to the early diagnosis of intraperitoneal injury. The ongoing exploration of indications for and advantages of these tests are discussed in more detail later in this chapter.

Within the changing total scenario of pediatric trauma, head injury is the primary determinant of outcome. Increasingly, solid visceral injury is managed nonoperatively. Abdominal intestinal trauma is infrequent and while a source of comorbidity, should rarely be the cause of mortality.

Diagnosis
History and Physical Examination

When possible, a detailed description of the mechanism of injury, the place and position in which the victim was found, details of transport (including times and need for extrication), and status of other victims provides clues about probable injury. For example, ejection from a vehicle increases the risk of injury by 300%.[3] Conversely, injuries out of proportion to or inconsistent with the history provided should raise the suspicion of child abuse.[4,5]

In most circumstances, a thorough physical examination may be all that is required for accurate evaluation of the abdomen. Skin bruising should raise the question of injury to underlying organs. If the pattern or distribution suggests abuse, photographic documentation is valuable. In specifically evaluating abdominal trauma, it should be noted if abdominal distention is relieved by a nasogastric tube. The quality of bowel sounds is meaningless, but their absence may have significance. Localized or diffuse tenderness, blood on rectal examination, and unstable pelvis or flank hematoma are highly significant findings.

For patients in whom examination is clearly normal or abnormal, few, if any, additional studies may be necessary. Additional diagnostic procedures are indicated only for those patients with indeterminate findings. Unfortunately, the accuracy of these procedures may be limited in cases with enteric injury.

Laboratory Evaluation

In all but the most trivial abdominal trauma, a complete blood count, blood urea nitrogen count, amylase and liver enzyme analysis, urinalysis, and plain abdominal x-rays for documentation are appropriate. While abnormal liver enzymes and urinalysis may be a clue to intra-abdominal injury, no test is particularly useful in diagnosing intestinal trauma.

Radiologic Evaluation

While plain films of the abdomen have long been recognized as having limited value in assessing acute intestinal injury, they serve several purposes. When it is present, free air simplifies decision making. In the absence of free air, value is derived from assessing bony injury and from documenting radiologic findings. Plain films may be underused in following the condition of patients with suspected abdominal trauma. Zahran and associates reviewed radiologic plain film techniques, which proved useful in demonstrating hollow viscus injuries in children. Using a combination of upright and decubitus films obtained after time for fluid collection, they were frequently able to recognize intraperitioneal fluid and air, notably in 6 of 7 jejunal perforations.[6] After reviewing 12 children with intestinal injury following blunt abdominal trauma, Mercer and coworkers recommend erect or decubitus films be performed every 6 to 8 hours for 48 hours to increase the diagnosis of free air.[7]

CT scanning has emerged rapidly as the most frequently used diagnostic procedure in trauma. Initially applied to adult trauma, its utility in pediatric trauma was quickly appreciated, if for no other reason than because it clearly documented extent of solid visceral injury treated without operation.

In a review of 100 children with blunt upper abdominal trauma, Kaufman and associates found that a CT scan is the single most useful imaging test available.[8] They did qualify this statement by saying that very few of their patients required operation, therefore confirmation of their findings was indirect. Of the many advantages of CT scan, the most important for pediatric abdominal trauma is that it is a noninvasive, nonorgan specific test that is particularly valuable in detecting injury to the liver and spleen, the most commonly injured organs. Disadvantages include a typical one-hour delay in obtaining the scan after it has been deemed necessary. There is significant variation in the quality of scans from different institutions, particularly when motion artifact is not eliminated. Other cited disadvantages include the cost of the procedure and the radiation exposure.

Patient selection for abdominal CT scanning is an unresolved debate. Clearly not all abdominal trauma requires a CT scan. Routine abdominal CT scans are not necessary in all children in whom a head CT is performed. Patient selection for abdominal CT scanning varies significantly between institutions. For the purposes of time and cost constraints some selection is necessary and is generally based on clinical evaluation and patterns of injury commonly associated with intra-abdominal trauma.

A recent study of abdominal CT scans performed on 65 children with a Glasgow Coma Score of less than 10 revealed 15 children with abdominal injuries.[9] While the authors interpreted this as demonstrating the value of CT scanning, no patients underwent immediate abdominal operations as a result of the CT scan. Documentation of intra-abdominal visceral injuries are important in assessing patient risk, deciding proper patient location in the hospital, and allocating blood and nursing resources, as well as diagnostic accuracy, even if there is no anticipation of an operation. Such diagnostic accuracy is beneficial should the patient experience clinical deterioration that later requires operation. In solid visceral injury, operative decisions are clinical, not radiologic.

The diagnostic accuracy of intestinal injury by abdominal CT scanning is generally considered to be limited.[10–13] To increase the accuracy of such scans in the presence of bowel perforation, oral contrast should be administered, preferably well before the scan. Donohue and associates reviewed 24 patients with bowel or mesenteric injury suspected by CT scan and concluded that CT scan is reliable in predicting injuries requiring repair using extraluminal gas or bowel wall hematomas accompanied by intraperitoneal fluid as operative indications.[14] While this implies an even greater specificity than is usually attributed to CT scan, it is significant coming from a trauma center that has performed 2000 abdominal scans in 6 years. In an editorial on CT scans, this same group said that in their emergency room 14 percent of patients with abdominal trauma have had CT scans, emphasizing that most patients are managed by clinical findings.[15]

Other radiologic studies are performed less frequently and for selected organ injuries. Ultrasound is infrequently used in situations of acute injury. Shaftan has speculated that in the future, it may become the emergency room procedure for identifying injuries.[16] It is arguably better than the CT scan for following pancreatic injuries, particularly pseudocysts, and is performed with lower monetary cost and radiation exposure level.

Upper gastrointestinal series is the procedure of choice to diagnose duodenal hematoma in the child with persistent vomiting after blunt epigastric trauma and no peritoneal signs. It is less accurate in identifying duodenal rupture.[17] The patient with potential bowel injury who is not improving as anticipated can be assessed later in the hospital course by sequential plain films, CT scanning, or DPL.

Lavage

The concept of sampling abdominal fluid to assess intraperitoneal injury is not new. The technique of peritoneal aspiration to identify intraperitoneal disease was described by Neuhof and Cohen in 1926.[18] In the ensuing years, improved survival of patients with operative treatment of abdominal trauma mandated this approach. Then, in the early 1960s, Shaftan described clinical criteria for deciding which patients required operation, and published good results in both operatively and nonoperatively treated patients.[2] The addition of lavage in 1965 increased the detection of intraperitoneal injury.[19]

By nearly unanimous agreement, a positive lavage is one with RBC >100,000/ml, WBC >500/ml, presence of stool, bile, amylase, or bacteria.[20,21] Using these criteria, DPL has a 98 percent accuracy in diagnosing intra-abdominal injury, with a false positive rate of 0.2 percent.[22] Presence of elevated amylase or 50,000–100,000 RBC/ml is a controversial indicator of injury, requiring operative intervention. Situations of increased diagnostic inaccuracy have been reported in patients with pelvic fractures, colonic injury, and gunshot wounds (GSW).[23–25] In a comparison of DPL and CT scan for evaluating blunt abdominal trauma, both tests had a high specificity, but DPL was more sensitive and less time consuming and costly.[26,27]

Open, semi-open and closed techniques have all been described for performing lavage. While the open technique, performed through a small infraumbilical incision carried down through the fascia, has no major associated complications, the closed technique has a 5 to 6 percent major complication rate.[28,29] The semi-open technique of Lazarus-Nelson, involving a small infraumbilical skin incision and a Seldinger technique for introducing the catheter, is reportedly without complications and most applicable to children.[30]

Diagnostic peritoneal lavage has proven to be a valuable tool in identifying adult patients with blunt abdominal trauma that requires laparotomy. In the pediatric population, the presence of intraperitoneal blood is not in itself an indication for laparotomy, as the majority of these patients are safely treated nonoperatively. In two reviews of DPL applied to children with blunt abdominal trauma, the use of RBC >100,000/ml as criteria indicating laparotomy led to unnecessary laparotomies in 34 to 67 percent of patients.[20,21] Further diagnostic studies were recommended to decrease the rate of laparotomy, but in many of these patients one wonders if DPL itself was unnecessary.

At CHM, we have developed a decision algorithim that combines clinical findings and selective use of abdominal CT scan and DPL.[22] This decreases the number of children receiving expensive or invasive procedures without sacrificing diagnostic accuracy. In this schema, DPL is used in three specific situations. The patient with apparent life-threatening extra-abdominal injury who requires emergent treatment for this condition undergoes DPL as the most expeditious way to assess abdominal injury. The technique is used in patients with negative or equivocal examinations, but with abdominal stab wounds suspected of penetrating the abdominal cavity. Finally, DPL has an important but limited role in the multiply injured patient for whom CT scan presumably excluded abdominal injury, but then develops unexplainable clinical deterioration.

Penetrating Injuries
Gunshot Wounds

While gunshot wounds (GSW) have been a more significant problem for the adult population, the incidence of pediatric GSWs is increasing, particularly in the adolescent population. Urban hospitals treat more GSWs than suburban or rural hospitals. The PTR reports a 3.4 percent overall incidence of GSWs, but the percentage of these that were abdominal is not stated. In an unpublished review of patients at CHM, GSWs were responsible for 8 percent of abdominal injuries. The circumstances surrounding pediatric GSWs differ from adult victims. The infant or toddler is usually the accidental victim of domestic violence. The older child is often shot when a gun she or he is playing with discharges. Children of all ages, particularly in urban settings, may be the victims of shootings when their guardians are involved in illicit activities. By adolescence, the circumstances are similar to adults with the victim also often the perpetrator of violence. An additional cause of adolescent GSWs is suicide, with most of the increasing incidence of suicide attributable to firearms.[34]

The approach to treatment of pediatric GSWs is fairly straightforward, with most surgeons agreeing that evidence of peritoneal penetration by the missile is sufficient indication for laparotomy. However, it should be noted that there may be a role in select cases for nonoperative management. In a large series of adults with penetrating abdominal injuries, McAlvanah and Shaftan observed 45 percent of patients with GSWs and had no morbidity or mortality in patients selected for nonoperative treatment.[35] Significant differences between children and adults make selective nonoperative treatment of abdominal GSWs more risky. The thinner abdominal wall of most children, compared to adults, means peritoneal penetration is much more likely to have occurred. The decreased incidence of pediatric GSWs also increases the chance of overlooking significant injuries with nonoperative treatment. Even strong advocates of nonoperative treatment of penetrating trauma qualify their stance by stating that for individuals or institutions not treating a high volume of such injuries, laparotomy is the more conservative treatment. A child who has recently sustained a GSW may not be able to cooperate with repeated physical examination or DPL. Therefore, our approach is to obtain two view abdominal x-rays in the stable child. If the bullet appears to be intraperitoneal or have followed an intraperitoneal trajectory, the patient is explored operatively. If the bullet has grazed the abdominal wall and the abdominal examination reveals no peritoneal signs, the patient is either admitted for observation or discharged from the emergency room.

In their review of abdominal GSWs, Valentine and associates routinely ex-

Table 11-1. Organ Injury in Penetrating Trauma

	Sinclair (1974)	Turnbull (1975)	Barlow (1982)	Valentine (1984)	CHM (1988)	Total
Small bowel	25	23	4	13	7	72
Stomach	10	18	4	4	5	41
Colon	17	14	4	7	4	46
Duodenum	3	9	2	2	0	16
Other Intra-abdominal	55	76	15	17	23	186

plored patients operatively and found that 19 percent had negative explorations.[36] The frequency of organ injury in gunshot and stab wounds in various series is shown in Table 11-1. The small bowel is the most frequently injured hollow viscus, and the liver and spleen are the most frequently injured solid organs. The significant complication rates in these series were low, but increased with injury from a large-caliber weapon or shotgut, number of organs injured, and delays in surgical correction of injuries.[37-41]

Stab Wounds

In the current approach to management of abdominal stab wounds there exists a common theme that a negative laparotomy is not a benign procedure. This reflects a significant change in attitudes, based on reviewing statistics of negative laparotomies. In a review of 245 trauma patients from Cook County Hospital, there was a 1.6 percent mortality, a 19 percent morbidity, and a 3 percent incidence of adhesive bowel obstruction.[42] Pediatric abdominal stab wound treatment has followed the practice in adults, so that selective exploration is the rule. The role of lavage in determining need for laparotomy remains controversial both in pediatric and adult series, with many clinicians believing that physical findings alone dictate need for laparotomy.[38,40,43-46] Proponents of peritoneal lavage claim that the rate of negative laparotomy can be reduced by lavage and that hospital courses can be shortened.[47,48]

Patients with abdominal stab wounds and peritoneal signs or hemodynamic instability warrant operation. Omental evisceration is another indication for exploration. It is difficult to reduce an omental evisceration in an awake child. Approximately 70 percent of these patients will also have significant visceral injury.[49,50] Lavage has a useful role in the patient with an equivocal examination, with the modifier that >100,000 RBC/ml alone may still not be an indication for laparotomy. Barlow and associates, in a review of pediatric stab wounds, employed selective management without lavage to patients with thoracoabdominal stab wounds.[40] Perhaps the 38 percent incidence of negative laparotomy could have been reduced by lavage.

Blunt Injuries

When children present after blunt trauma with peritonitis or hypotension unrelieved by fluid resuscitation, the decision to operate is clear. The real problem is the child who is being managed nonoperatively and who develops a fever on the second hospital day, has a prolonged ileus, or has worsening pain. Depending on the clinician's index of suspicion, either further diagnostic studies may be helpful or laparotomy is undertaken. Both the early and late indications for abdominal exploration must be clear to minimize delays in the decision to operate (Table 11-2).

Historically, the diagnosis of small bowel injuries has frequently been delayed

Table 11-2. Indications for Abdominal Exploration

Acute	Late
Refractory hypotension	Peritonitis
Peritonitis	Contrast extravasation on CT
	or upper gastric series
Free air	Free air
Positive DPL*	Positive DPL*

* RBC >100,000 is not in itself considered indication for laparotomy. WBC >500, + gram stain, culture, bile, or GI contents constitute positive indications.

because of the late appearance of free air. This may still be the case occasionally. If at any time after initial assessment and management, repetitive examinations or clinical course raises the spectre of occult intestinal injury, repeat plain abdominal x-rays should be obtained. In the absence of free air, DPL can be valuable. While we have elected to avoid nonselective DPL in all abdominal trauma, it can provide a diagnosis of intestinal injury prior to the appearance of free air on plain films. The increasing experience and success with the nonoperative treatment of splenic and, subsequently, of hepatic injuries in children places an increasing responsibility on the clinician to recognize intestinal injury. It has the advantages of speed, bedside application, and in lesions distal to the duodenum, greater accuracy than the CT scan with contrast. The CT scan with oral and intravenous contrast is noninvasive, has good reliability in duodenal injuries, and accurately assesses solid visceral injury, the retroperitoneum, and localized fluid collections.

Such delayed DPL avoids unnecessary use for very low frequency injuries, can shorten the traditional delays of a plain film diagnosis of free air, and avoids unnecessary laparotomy. Such an approach does place great importance on the clinician and repetitive assessments. Fortunately, even with delayed operative intervention for enteric injury, outcome is good.[51] An example of the utility of DPL is a 4-year-old who was treated with initial volume resuscitation and mechanical ventilation for severe closed head injury, rib fractures, pulmonary contusion, Class III hepatic laceration, and sexual abuse. Fever and some increased abdominal distention on the second hospital day precipitated a DPL that produced few white cells and no bacteria with subsequently sterile cultures. Laparotomy was avoided and discharge occurred 12 days after injury.

Specific Organ Injury
Stomach

The incidence of gastric injury is low and dependent on the mechanism of injury. In blunt abdominal trauma, gastric rupture varies from no incidence to 1.7 percent.[29,52] In the series of penetrating injuries, the incident of gastric injuries varied from 7 to 13 percent.[37,38,41,53] While it has been stated that gastric injury is more common in children than in adults, comparison of series fail to confirm this.[54] In contrast with other hollow viscus injuries, gastric perforation may be recognized by the presence of free air on upright films of the abdomen. The physiology of gastric rupture relates to intramural rather than intraluminal pressure and to rapid increases in intra-abdominal and intragastric pressures.[52] In contrast to adults, where the lesser curvature is the more frequent site of rupture, the greater curvature is more frequently the site of perforation in children.[55] Isolated gastric injury is rarely associated with hypotension and is treated by the removal of particulate debris from the peritoneal cavity and closure of the defect. Debridement of wound edges may be appropriate. Significant complications are unusual, but include subphrenic abscess and gastric fistula. Injury to the spleen, liver, and pancreas should be sought specifically at the time of exploration.

Duodenum

Although duodenal injury is relatively uncommon, it receives more attention because it is associated with significant morbidity and mortality and operative treatment varies. Because of its protected position, the duodenum is injured in zero to 6 percent of patients with penetrating abdominal trauma.[37,38,52,53] While the incidence of duodenal injury following blunt trauma is generally quoted as 1 to 2 percent, in their exhaustive review of patients admitted for blunt trauma, Fischer and associates documented a 0.1 percent incidence in children and a 0.5 percent incidence in adults.[1]

Duodenal injury is most commonly the result of a direct blow to the epigastrium. The classic pediatric injury is the duodenal hematoma with epigastric bruising that results from a handlebar injury. Other mechanisms include baseballs, fists, falls, or minor epigastric trauma in a child with an underlying coagulopathy such as hemophilia or leukemia. Motor vehicle accidents (MVA) are also a common cause.

While seatbelts have decreased the mortality from MVA, at least one study reports an increased incidence of gastrointestinal injuries.[56] Unfortunately, this study did not differentiate belt restraints from shoulder harnesses. Agran and associates examined injuries sustained by children using vehicle seatbelts rather than child safety seats, and found that mechanism of injury changed with the age or, more likely, the size of the child. Abdominal injuries are more likely in the the 4 to 9 year age group. Restraints may increase intraluminal pressure at points of fixation and increase the possibility of duodenal injury.[57] An unusual example is an 8-year-old child, restrained in a MVA, with critical head injury and showing initially normal clinical and CT evaluation of the abdomen. Central nervous system (CNS) recovery was very prolonged and feeding intolerance progressed long after injury. A CT study with intragastric contrast revealed a duodenal intussusception, which was reduced at laparotomy (Fig. 11-1).

The radiologic limitations in the diagnosis of duodenal injury have been discussed previously. The upper GI series is the superior technique for the diagnosis

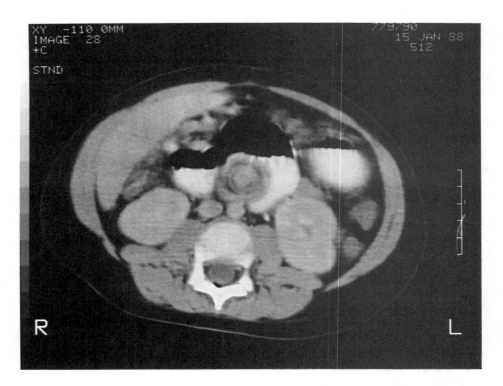

Figure 11-1. CT scan with oral and IV contrast in patient with post-traumatic duodenal intussusception.

of duodenal hematoma and can be selected because the child has minimal peritoneal findings and a characteristic history. The classic finding in adults is the "coiled spring or stacked coin" appearance. In the majority of these children, this classic sign is less clear and only partial duodenal obstruction is seen. In the patient with more significant peritoneal findings, the CT scan is generally performed and should be accompanied by oral contrast. The limitations of the upper GI series are thereby minimized.

The surgical principles for treating duodenal injuries are the same in children as in adults. For the purposes of discussing these injuries, Lucas and Ledgerwood's classification is useful.[58] Class 1 and class 2 are incomplete and complete duodenal perforation, respectively, without pancreatic injuries. Class 3 includes minor pancreatic injuries and Class 4 is associated with major pancreatic injuries. Duodenal hematomas are Class 1 injuries. The typical patient has suffered blunt abdominal trauma and may have localized pain, but may not seek attention or the diagnosis suspected until the later onset of vomiting. Touloukian has outlined a useful management schema for these patients, consisting of early upper gastric series, NG decompression, and total parenteral nutrition (TPN). Patients without pancreatic injury responded to this therapy and were discharged within one week. In this series, even the patients with pancreatic injuries were treated nonoperatively, but required longer hospitalization.[59] In an extensive review of the literature, Jewett and associates found all cases were secondary to blunt abdominal trauma, with pancreatitis the most frequent associated injury (21%).[60] Because child abuse can be a cause of pancreatitis, particularly in children less than 3 years old, a careful history with social service evaluation is warranted in suspect cases.[61] Surgical treatment of this lesion is associated with longer hospitalization and a 15 percent rate of complications, and therefore should be reserved for the rare patient who fails to resolve or appears to have associated injuries requiring laparotomy (Fig. 11-2). When laparotomy is performed, evacuation of the hematoma with repair of the serosa is all that is necessary.

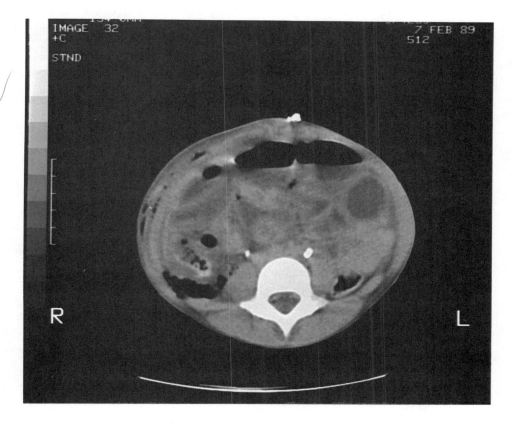

Figure 11-2. CT scan with oral and IV contrast for duodenal hematoma with complete duodenal obstruction secondary to abuse. Note lack of contrast in small bowel and edema in bowel wall. Upper gastric test series filled only the stomach. Oral feedings resumed two and one-half weeks after nonoperative management.

Class 2 duodenal injuries are best treated by simple one-layer or two-layer repair with drainage.[62–64] Treatment of Class 3 and Class 4 injuries is more controversial and regardless of the procedure chosen is associated with significant morbidity and mortality. Surgical options for these injuries include primary repair and drainage with or without tube decompression, onlay serosal patches, resection and anastomosis, duodenal diverticularization, pyloric exclusion, or pancreaticoduodenectomy. Review of published series shows there to be no consensus as to appropriate management, but several facts emerge. When a duodenal fistula forms, the mortality may be as high as 42 percent.[63,65] Diverting intestinal flow from a severely injured duodenum by tube decompression or diverticularization decreases fistulization.[68,69,78,79] Pancreaticoduodenectomy is rarely needed for trauma and because it is associated with a mortality rate as high as 40 percent, it should be reserved for cases in which no other treatment is feasible.[62,70] Blunt duodenal trauma is associated with a higher morbidity and mortality and a more frequent delay in diagnosis than penetrating injuries.[71] In a recently reported series of pediatric pancreaticoduodenal injuries, Pokorny and coworkers successfully treated 9 children with major pancreatic injuries. Of 7 patients treated with duodenorrhaphy, 4 developed fistulae, all of which closed without secondary surgical intervention.[64]

Small Bowel. Penetrating abdominal trauma in adults is associated with a 30 percent incidence of small bowel injuries.[53] Because penetrating injuries are much less common in children, the incidence is less clearly defined. Over a 5-year period at CHM, 50 children had penetrating injuries out of 277 torso trauma admissions, an incidence of 18 percent.[41] There were only 5 patients with small bowel perforations and 2 small bowel eviscerations. Small bowel injuries are less common in both children and adults with blunt trauma. While Blaisdell quotes a 9 percent small bowel injury rate for adults,[53] Fischer reported a 25 percent rate of gastrointestinal disruption in adults requiring surgery. Of 1275 children admitted in Fischer's series, 46 underwent laparotomy and only 3 had gastrointestinal disruption.[1]

In a review of blunt intestinal trauma, Dauterive and coworkers found peritoneal lavage to be diagnostic in 95 percent of patients. Associated intra-abdominal injuries occurred in 43 percent of patients and extra-abdominal injuries in 78 percent.[72] In contrast to this series with a low incidence of duodenal injury, Donahue and coworkers reported 50 percent of patients with intestinal injury following blunt trauma had duodenal injury.[73] Regardless of the series, the treatment of extraduodenal small bowel injury is straightforward. Primary repair is suitable for most stab wounds or blunt injuries involving less than one third of circumference of the bowel. Resection and reanastomosis is appropriate for most gunshot wounds, mesenteric vascular injuries, or disruption of more than one third of bowel circumference. The complication rate is generally low, is usually infectious, and is greatly increased when the diagnosis of intestinal injury is delayed more than 24 hours.

The presentation of pediatric patients with small bowel injury is similar to that of adults, with pain being the most frequent symptom. Delay in diagnosis remains a problem because of the infrequency of occurrence, delay in appearance of free air on x-ray, and the fact that most blunt trauma is now treated nonoperatively.[51,74,75] Only 40 percent of patients in Kako and associates' series demonstrated free air.[75] As previously mentioned, repeat multiple-view abdominal plain films can be quite helpful in detecting retroperitoneal gas collections or free air that was not present on initial x-rays. Children not following the expected course after blunt abdominal trauma deserve aggressive evaluation as discussed earlier. Kako and associates' reported 8 percent mortality and 35 percent complication rates indicate that although small bowel injuries may be uncommon, they must not be overlooked.[75] In our experience, such mortality is an indication of associated injuries.

Specific comment regarding small bowel injury in abused children is appropriate. While central upper abdominal injuries to pancreas, liver and spleen predominate, small bowel injury does occur. It is highly characteristic in that there is intramural hematoma and avulsion of the gut from the mesentery with or without perforation, as seen in Figure 11-3. The clinical characteristics that should suggest abuse are a history of illness incompatible with the severity of physical findings; parental evasiveness; skin findings of bruising, whip marks or cigarette burns; and fractures of varied ages and patterns on long bone x-ray films. An example is a

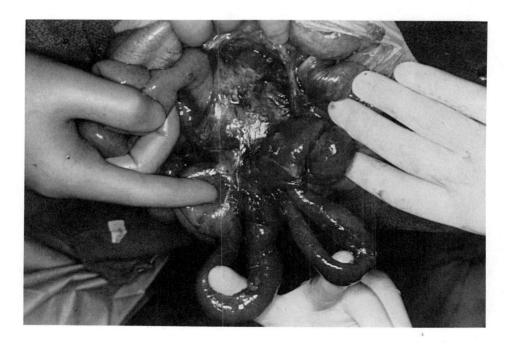

Figure 11-3. Mesenteric avulsion, serosal degloving injury and sealed perforation in blunt trauma from child abuse.

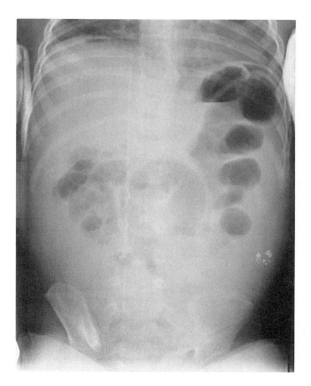

Figure 11-4. Plain film of an abused 2-year-old reveals ileus and free air. Tibial and metacarpal fractures were noted on skeletal films.

two-year-old girl with hypotension, fever, and peritoneal findings, in whom initial plain films (Fig. 11-4) revealed ileus and a small amount of free air. The only history was that she "got sick last night." Free air may be seen in this setting because of parental delay in evaluation. Laparotomy revealed several areas of avulsion of the jejunum from the mesentery and a sealed perforation.

Colon

Colonic injuries occur less frequently than small bowel injuries both in blunt and penetrating trauma. In adult series, the incidence is 4 percent and 9 percent, respectively.[53] In combined series of both penetrating and blunt injuries in children, the incidence of colon injuries is 10 percent.[76] Treatment of these injuries has changed from mandatory colostomy for all transmural injuries to selective colostomy to predominantly primary closure.

Because of the relative infrequency of these injuries and the increasing use of nonoperative treatment of blunt trauma, the diagnosis is often delayed. Emergent CT scan is unreliable for detecting hollow viscus injury.[77] Delayed scan may be helpful when the clinical situation is confusing. Indeed, in a patient recently treated at CHM, a degloving injury of the sigmoid with no perforation and ileocecal perforation was suggested by increased soft tissue densities in these regions on CT scan (Fig. 11-5). Probably more helpful in these cases would be lavage which would be expected to show both bacteria and elevated WBC counts.

The adult literature on the management of penetrating colon injuries serves as the guideline for managing these injuries in children because no equivalent pediatric series exist. In a recent review of unintentional pediatric firearm deaths, 57 percent were secondary to handguns, 43 percent secondary to long guns, and 33 percent died immediately, so it is a safe assumption that children also sustain serious firearm injury.[78] Stone and Fabian performed the first randomized prospective study comparing primary closure with exteriorization. With the exclusion of patients who were in profound shock, had more than two intra-abdominal organs injured, and had gross fecal contamination, patients undergoing primary repair had decreased morbidity and shorter hospitalizations.[79] In a more recent review of 727 patients with colonic injuries undergoing primary repair, exteriorized repair, or colostomy, Burch and associates found decreased abscess formation, fecal fistula, and mortality in patients treated by primary repair.[80] The old concept that primary closure of right colon injuries is safer than left colon injuries has also been

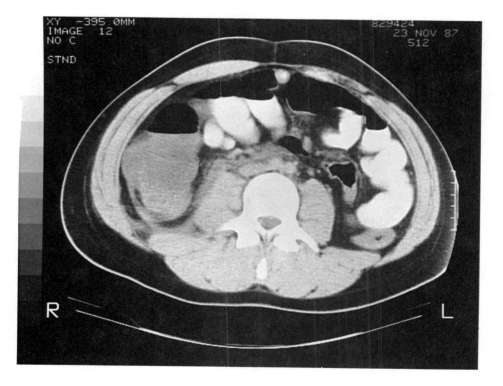

Figure 11-5. CT scan with oral contrast three days after seatbelt injury in MVA shows ileus, thickened bowel, and abnormal fluid collection lateral to cecum. Initial studies were normal.

refuted.[81,82] There does seem to be a consensus that the most severely injured patients are treated most safely by colostomy or exteriorized repair.[83,84] While exteriorization seems to be accompanied by a higher complication rate than colostomy in these patients, some surgeons advocate this type of repair.[85]

Rectum

Most pediatric rectal injuries are "straddle" injuries. The typical patient presents with local pain, bruising, and bleeding and is extremely anxious and difficult to examine. For this reason, it is our practice to perform examination under anesthesia with sigmoidoscopy and vaginoscopy whenever the diagnosis is considered. Mucosal or partial-thickness injury can be treated with evacuation of the rectum and observation. If a full-thickness injury is detected, it is repaired and proximal colostomy is performed. When injury is associated with extensive fecal contamination, devitalized tissue, or results from a high-velocity missile, rectal washout and placement of presacral drains is indicated.[85,86] With severe injuries, careful evaluation for associated injuries is mandatory. If a urethral injury is suspected, a retrograde urethrogram should be performed prior to any instrumentation. Genitourinary tract and small bowel injuries are the most frequently associated injuries.[85,87]

Summary

When laparotomy is performed on children for abdominal trauma and intestinal injury is found, the operative principles followed are the same as those used for adults. Significant differences exist between children and adults in mechanisms of injury, evaluation, and number of patients requiring operation. Children sustain more blunt trauma at lower velocity and have a lower incidence of hollow viscus injury. Penetrating trauma is less common. While CT scan and peritoneal lavage have increased the ability to diagnose organ injury, both have limitations, particularly in detecting intestinal injury. Careful physical examination and clinical judgement still remain the most reliable indicators of which children require operation.

References

1. Fischer RP, Miller-Crotchett P, Reed RL: Gastrointestinal disruption: The hazard of nonoperative management in adults with blunt abdominal injury. J Trauma 28:1445, 1988
2. Shaftan GW: Indications for operation in abdominal trauma. Amer J Surg 99:657, 1960
3. Committee on Trauma: Advanced Trauma Life Support Course. Chicago, American College of Surgeons, 1989
4. Kempe CH, Silverman FN, Steele BF et al: The battered child syndrome. JAMA 181:205, 1962
5. Ledbetter DV, Hatch EF, Feldman KW et al: Diagnostic and surgical implications of child abuse. Arch Surg 123:1101, 1988

6. Zahran M, Eklof O, Thomasson B: Blunt abdominal trauma and hollow viscus injury in children: The diagnostic value of plain radiography. Pediatr Radiol 14:304, 1984

7. Mercer S, Legrand L, Stringel G et al: Delay in diagnosing gastrointestinal injury after blunt abdominal trauma in chidlren. Can J Surg 28:138, 1985

8. Kaufman RA, Towbin R, Babcock DS et al: Upper abdominal trauma in children: Imaging evaluation. AJR 142:449, 1984

9. Beaver BL, Colombani PM, Fal A et al: The efficacy of computed tomography in evaluating abdominal injuries in children with major head trauma. J Pediatr Surg 22:1117, 1987

10. Karp MP, Cooney DR, Berger PE et al: The role of computed tomography in the evaluation of blunt abdominal trauma in children. J Pediatr Surg 16:316, 1981

11. Peitzman AB, Makaroun MS, Slasky S et al: Prospective study of computed tomography in initial management of blunt abdominal trauma. J Trauma 26:585, 1986

12. Kane, NM, Cronan JJ, Dorfman GS et al: Pediatric abdominal trauma: Evaluation by computed tomography. Pediatr 82:11, 1988

13. Cook DE, Walsh JW, Vick CW et al: Upper abdominal trauma: Pitfalls in CT diagnosis. Radiol 159:65, 1986

14. Donohue JH, Federle MP, Griffiths BG et al: Computed tomography in the diagnosis of blunt intestinal and mesenteric injuries. J Trauma 27:11, 1987

15. Trunkey D, Federle MP: Computed tomography in perspective. J Trauma 26:660, 1986

16. Shaftan GW: Abdominal trauma management in America. Bulletin Am Coll Surg 74:21, 1989

17. Kelly G, Norton L, Moore G et al: The continuing challenge of duodenal injuries. J Trauma 18:160, 1978

18. Neuhof H, Cohen I: Abdominal puncture in the diagnosis of acute intraperitoneal disease. Ann Surg 83:454, 1926

19. Root HD, Hauser CW, McKinley CR et al: Diagnostic peritoneal lavage. Surgery 57:633, 1965

20. Thal ER, Shires GT: Peritoneal lavage in blunt abdominal trauma. Am J Surg 125:64, 1973

21. Parvin S, Smith DE, Asher WM: Effectiveness of peritoneal lavage. Ann Surg 181:255, 1975

22. Fischer RP, Beverlin BC, Engrav LH et al: Diagnostic peritoneal lavage: Fourteen years and 2,586 patients later. Am J Surg 136:701, 1978

23. Hubbard SG, Bivins BA, Sachatello CR et al: Diagnostic errors with peritoneal lavage in patients with pelvic fractures. Arch Surg 114:844, 1979

24. Obeid FN, Sorensen V, Vincent G et al: Inaccuracy of diagnostic peritoneal lavage in penetrating colonic trauma. Arch Surg 119:906, 1984

25. Thal ER, May RA, Bessinger D: Peritoneal lavage. Arch Surg 115:430, 1980

26. Marx JA, Moore EE, Jorden RC et al: Limitations of computed tomography in the evaluation of acute abdominal trauma: A prospective comparison with diagnostic peritoneal lavage. J Trauma 25:933, 1985

27. Kearney PA, Vahey T, Burney RE et al: Computed tomography and diagnostic peritoneal lavage in blunt abdominal trauma. Arch Surg 124:344, 1989

28. Moore JB, Moore EE, Markovchick VJ et al: Diagnostic peritoneal lavage for abdominal trauma: Superiority of the open technique at the infraumbilical ring. J Trauma 21:570, 1981

29. Pachter HL, Hofstetter SR: Open and percutaneous paracentesis and lavage for abdominal trauma. Arch Surg 116:318, 1981
30. Lazarus HM, Nelson JA: The surgeon at work: A technique for peritoneal lavage without risk or complication. Surg Gynecol Obstet 149:889, 1979
31. Powell RW, Green JB, Ochsner MG et al: Peritoneal lavage in pediatric patients sustaining blunt abdominal trauma: A reappraisal. J Trauma 27:6, 1987
32. Rothenberg S, Moore EE, Marx JA et al: Selective management of blunt abdominal trauma in children: The triage role of peritoneal lavage. J Trauma 27:1101, 1987
33. Long JA, Klein MD: Trauma in infants and children: Special considerations. In Walt AJ, Wilson RF (eds): Management of Trauma: Pitfalls and Practice. (in press)
34. Morbidity and Mortality Weekly Report 36:531, 1987
35. McAlvanah MJ, Shaftan GW: Selective conservatism in penetrating abdominal wounds: A continuing reappraisal. J Trauma 18:206, 1978
36. Valentine J, Blocker S, Chang J: Gunshot injuries in children. J Trauma 24:952, 1984
37. Sinclair MC, Moore TC: Major surgery for abdominal and thoracic trauma in childhood and adolescence. J Pediatr Surg 9:155, 1974
38. Tunell WP, Knost J, Nance FC: Penetrating abdominal injuries in children and adolescents. J Trauma 15:720, 1975
39. Barlow B, Niemirska M, Gandhi RP: Ten years' experience with pediatric gunshot wounds. J Pediatr Surg 17:927, 1982
40. Barlow B, Niemirska M, Gandhi RP: Stab wounds in children. J Pediatr Surg 18:926, 1983
41. Long JA, Philippart AI: Penetrating injuries in children. In Buntain WL (ed): Management of Pediatric Trauma. WB Saunders (in press)
42. Lowe RJ, Boyd DR, Folk FA et al: The negative laparotomy for abdominal trauma. J Trauma 12:853, 1972
43. Shorr RM, Gottlieb MM, Webb K et al: Selective management of abdominal stab wounds. Arch Surg 123:1141, 1988
44. Nance FC, Wennar MH, Johnson LW et al: Surgical judgment in the management of penetrating wounds of the abdomen: Experience with 2212 patients. Ann Surg 179:639, 1974
45. de Lacy AM, Pera M, Garcia-Valdecasas JC et al: Management of penetrating abdominal stab wounds. Br J Surg 75:231, 1988
46. Demetriades D, Rabinowitz B: Selective conservative management of penetrating abdominal wounds: A prospective study. Br J Surg 71:92, 1984
47. Thal ER: Evaluation of peritoneal lavage and local exploration in lower chest and abdominal stab wounds. J Trauma 17:642, 1977
48. Thompson JS, Moore EE, van Duzer-Moore S et al: The evolution of abdominal stab wound management. J Trauma 20:478, 1980
49. Granson MA, Donovan AJ: Abdominal stab wound with omental evisceration. Arch Surg 188:57, 1983
50. Burnweit CA, Thal ER: Significance of omental evisceration in abdominal stab wounds. Am J Surg 152:670, 1986
51. Cobb LM, Vinocur CD, Wagner CW et al: Intestinal perforation due to blunt trauma in children in an era of increased nonoperative treatment. J Trauma 26:461, 1986
52. Yajko RD, Seydel F, Trimble C: Rupture of the stomach from blunt abdominal trauma. J Trauma 15:178, 1975

53. Blaisdell FW: General assessment, resuscitation and exploration of penetraing and blunt abdominal injury. In Trauma Management, vol 1. (Abdominal Trauma), p 1. New York, Thieme-Stratten, 1982

54. Eichelberger, MR, Randolph JG: Abdominal trauma. In Pediatric Surgery, vol 1, 4th ed, p 154. Chicago, Yearbook Medical Publishers, 1986

55. McCormick WF: Rupture of the stomach in children: Review of the literature and report of seven cases. AMA Arch Pathol 67:416, 1959

56. Denis R, Allard M, Atlas H et al: Changing trends with abdominal injury in seatbelt wearers. J Trauma 23:1007, 1983

57. Agran PF, Dunkle DE, Winn DG: Injuries to a sample of seatbelted children evaluated and treated in a hospital emergency room. J Trauma 27:58, 1987

58. Lucas CE, Ledgerwood AM: Factors influencing outcome after blunt duodenal injury. J Trauma 15:839, 1975

59. Touloukian RJ: Protocol for the nonoperative treatment of obstructing duodenal hematoma during childhood. Am J Surg 145:330, 1983

60. Jewett TC, Caldarola V, Karp MP et al: Intramural hematoma of the duodenum. Arch Surg 123:54, 1988

61. Zieglar DW, Long JA, Philippart AI et al: Pancreatitis in childhood. Ann Surg 207:257, 1988

62. Synder WH, Weigeit JA, Watkins et al: The surgical management of duodenal trauma. Arch Surg 115:422, 1980

63. Flint LM, McCoy M, Richardson JD et al: Duodenal injury. Ann Surg 191:697, 1980

64. Pokorny WJ, Brandt, ML, Harberg FJ: Major duodenal injuries in children: Diagnosis, operative management, and outcome. J Pediatr Surg 21:613, 1986

65. Hasson NE, Stern D, Moss GS: Penetrating duodenal trauma. J Trauma 24:471, 1984

66. Stone HH, Fabian TC: Management of duodenal wounds. J Trauma 19:334, 1979

67. Feliciano DV, Martin TD, Cruse PA et al: Management of combined pancreatico-duodenal injuries. Ann Surg 205:673, 1987

68. Berne CJ, Donovan AJ, White EJ et al: Duodenal "diverticulization" for duodenal and pancreatic injury. Am J Surg 127:503, 1974

69. Vaughan, GD, Frazier OH, Graham DY et al: The use of pyloric exclusion in the management of severe duodenal injuries. Am J Surg 134:785, 1977

70. Oreskovich MR, Carrico CJ: Pancreaticoduodenectomy for trauma: A viable option? Am J Surg 147:618, 1984

71. Levison MA, Petersen SR, Sheldon GF et al: Duodenal trauma: Experience of a trauma center. J Trauma 24:475, 1984

72. Dauterive AH, Flancbaum L, Cox EF: Blunt intestinal trauma. Ann Surg 201:198, 1985

73. Donohue JH, Crass RA, Trunkey DD: The management of duodenal and other small intestinal trauma. World J Surg 9:904, 1985

74. Dickinson SJ, Shaw A, Santulli TV: Rupture of the gastrointestinal tract in children by blunt trauma. Surg Gynecol Obstet 131:655, 1970

75. Kakos GS, Grosfeld JL, Morse TS: Small bowel injuries in children after blunt abdominal trauma. Ann Surg 174:238, 1971

76. Welch KJ: Abdominal injuries. In The Injured Child, p 155. Chicago, Yearbook Medical Publishers, 1979

77. Kuhn JP: Diagnostic imaging for the evaluation of abdominal trauma in children. Pediatr Clin North Am 32:1327, 1985

78. Wintemute GJ, Kraus JP, Teret SJ et al: Unintentional firearm deaths in California. J Trauma 29:457, 1989

79. Stone HH, Fabian TC: Management of perforating colon trauma. Ann Surg 190:431, 1979

80. Burch JM, Gevirtzman BS, Jordan GL et al: The injured colon. Ann Surg 203:701, 1986

81. Flint, LM, Vitale GC, Richardson JD et al: The injured colon. Ann Surg 193:619, 1981

82. Thompson JS, Moore EE, Moore JB: Comparison of penetrating injuries of the right and left colon. Ann Surg 193:414, 1981

83. Adkins RB, Zinkle PK, Waterhause G: Penetrating colon trauma. J Trauma 24:491, 1984

84. Cook A, Levine BA, Rusing T et al: Traditional treatment of colon injuries. Arch Surg 119:591, 1984

85. Trunkey D, Hays RJ, Shires GT: Management of rectal trauma. J Trauma 13:411, 1973

86. Tuggle D, Huber PJ: Management of rectal trauma. Am J Surg 148:806, 1984

87. Robertson HD, Ray JE, Ferrari BT et al: Management of rectal trauma. Surg Gynecol Obstet 154:161, 1982

CHAPTER 12

Management of Blunt Pancreatic Trauma in Children

C. A. Burnweit and R. M. Filler

*T*he pancreas is injured in less than 10 percent of patients hospitalized for blunt abdominal trauma.[1] Because the pancreas occupies a relatively protected position in the retroperitoneum, children who present with a pancreatic injury usually have been victims of severe trauma. Morbidity and prolonged hospitalization are common after blunt and penetrating pancreatic trauma. Mortality figures of up to 19 percent have been reported in several large series that include victims of all ages.[2-4] These data may not be completely accurate for the childhood population.

Injury to the pancreas in children is usually caused by the organ's compression against the rigid vertebral column. Boys are more likely than girls to sustain pancreatic trauma.[5-8] Pancreatic injury is commonly seen after bicycle handle-bar injuries, falls, child abuse, and motor vehicle accidents, especially in those children restrained by simple lap belts.[3,5-8]

Controversy exists regarding the optimal treatment for pancreatic injury. Much of the surgical literature has supported early operative intervention, both in adult and pediatric series.[1-8] In our experience, however, most children have been treated without initial surgery with equally good results.

In the past 7 years we have seen 29 children with significant pancreatic injury following blunt trauma. The purpose of this report is to outline our plan of diagnosis and management of blunt pancreatic injuries and their sequelae and to compare our experience with the literature.

Diagnosis

Most children who have sustained forces great enough to injure the pancreas have signs and symptoms referable to the abdomen after the injury. In some cases, however, the symptoms may be subtle and medical attention is not sought immediately. Other patients have been sent home after initial medical evaluation, only to return several days later. In our recent series, 38 percent of patients with serious pancreatic trauma were seen more than 24 hours after the initial injury. Results from other centers also suggest that as many as half of pancreatic injuries present late.[4,8,9] Table 12-1 lists the causes of injury for the children in our series.

Initial management of the acutely injured child follows the principles set down by all modern trauma manuals and the Advanced Life Trauma Support (ATLS) course. Airway compromise and hemodynamic instability are treated rapidly. A complete physical exam is performed to rule out other injuries. A few patients who have sustained abdominal injury have obvious clinical signs of massive intra-abdominal bleeding and are taken directly to the operating room for laparotomy. However, the majority of children who present with multi-system or major abdominal trauma do not have hemodynamic compromise. Further evaluation with a selected diagnostic battery of tests is indicated. We routinely perform chest, pelvis, and lateral cervical spine radiographs and send blood for complete blood cell-count (CBC), liver function, and amylase determinations.

Like most other pediatric centers, we do not perform abdominal taps or peritoneal lavage routinely. This technique is invasive, painful, and difficult to perform in an uncooperative youngster. In addition, serial physical exams become more difficult after lavage and lavage may miss injuries to retroperitoneal structures such as the duodenum and pancreas. Furthermore, we do not believe that the presence of blood in the peritoneum *per se* is an indication for surgery.[10,11] In special circumstances, however, such as the unconscious child taken immediately to the operating room for the treatment of a life-threatening neurological or peripheral vascular injury, peritoneal lavage is employed.

We rely on computed tomographic (CT) scans with and without contrast to evaluate the status of the abdominal viscera. A CT scan identifies spleen and liver injuries accurately, evaluates the integrity and function of the urinary tract, and is extremely useful for the diagnosis of pancreatic injuries. Pancreatic injury can be inferred when the pancreas is swollen or disrupted or when there is a collection

Table 12-1. Cause of Pediatric Blunt Pancreatic Injuries in a Seven-Year Period

Cause	Number
Bicyle accidents	9
Pedestrian-MVA	5
Child abuse	2
Hockey injury	3
Snowmobile injury	3
Fall from height	3
Other	4

of fluid in the lesser sac. The false negative rate of CT scan for detection of pancreatic trauma is less than 1 percent.[12]

Abdominal utrasonography has not been as accurate as CT in the complete evaluation of the abdominal viscera after trauma. It is, however, extremely useful and reliable to follow a pancreatic injury with or without a pseudocyst.

Endoscopic retrograde cholangiopancreatography (ERCP) is not indicated for the child with an acute pancreatic injury. This study may be useful for the evaluation of chronic pancreatitis or for a persistent pseudocyst following abdominal trauma. Occasionally a ductal injury that cannot be demonstrated using other modalities will be evident when contrast study is performed of the duct of Wirsung.

Serum amylase elevations are sometimes difficult to interpret in the face of acute trauma. While all but 2 of the 29 patients with pancreatic trauma in our current series had an elevated serum amylase (mean 712±743 IU, range 59 to 2800 IU), similar levels can be seen in those with bowel or facial trauma. Although high amylase values suggest a pancreatic injury, they need to be viewed in the context of all clinical findings.

Clinical Experience at the Hospital for Sick Children

We have treated 29 children for blunt pancreatic injuries in the Hospital for Sick Children (HSC) over the past 7 years. In all cases, the diagnosis of pancreatic injury was confirmed by one or more of the following methods: ultrasound, CT scan, intraoperative inspection, and post-mortem examination. Twenty five children received initial treatment at this hospital and 4 were referred to us after surgery elsewhere.

Five of the 25 children with pancreatic injury seen first at our hospital underwent emergency operation for signs of peritonitis or because of uncontrolled hemorrhage (Fig. 12-1). In addition to the pancreatic lesion, each child had at least one other major intra-abdominal injury that was the principal indication for surgery. Four patients had bowel injuries, 2 had diaphragmatic ruptures, and 1 had an hepatic avulsion. The pancreatic lesion was treated in only 1 patient, in whom distal pancreatectomy was performed because of a completely transected gland. No specific therapy for the pancreatic lesion was undertaken in the other 4. The only 2 deaths in our series occurred among these 5 patients. A 2-year-old boy, who had fallen 9 stories, died in the operating room of combined head, pulmonary and hepatic injuries. A second child, who had been crushed in a garbage compressor, died 20 hours post-operatively from progressive respiratory failure. The pancreatic injuries contributed to neither death. The remaining 3 children recovered without complications.

The remaining 20 children evaluated initially at our facilities were managed nonoperatively (Fig. 12-2). Eight recovered without complication and were dis-

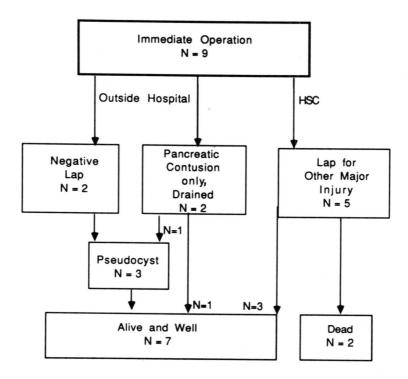

Figure 12-1. Outcome of children with pancreatic trauma who received early operation.

charged after a mean hospital stay of 21 days (range, 2–41 days). Pseudocysts developed in 11 of the other 12 children and pancreatitis occurred in 1. This last child had endoscopic retrograde pancreatography 3 months after trauma and was found to have a mid-duct stricture with distal ductal dilatation and a small pseudocyst. A distal pancreatectomy was curative. Seven of the 11 (64%) pancreatic pseudocysts resolved with bowel rest and total parenteral nutrition (TPN) after an average hospitalization of 28 days (range, 15–42 days). Drainage procedures (as noted below) were necessary for the 4 pseudocysts that did not resolve with nonoperative therapy.

Four boys who underwent laparotomy elsewhere (See Fig. 12-1) were transferred to our hospital for post-operative care. In two, a pancreatic contusion was noted as the sole injury and the lesser sac was drained. In one case, the drain was removed and the child was discharged nine days after injury without complications. In the other case, a pseudocyst developed. In the other two boys, no pancreatic injury was identified and no drains were left in the abdomen; pseudocysts developed in both cases.

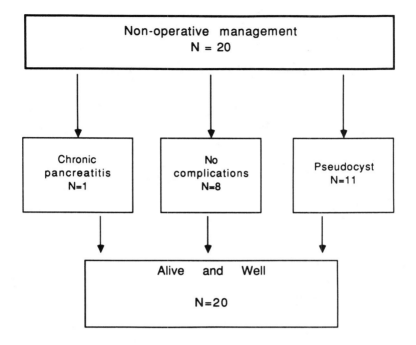

Figure 12-2. Outcome of children with pancreatic trauma who were treated initially with medical therapy.

Pancreatic Pseudocysts

Pancreatic pseudocyst is the most commonly encountered complication following pancreatic trauma in the pediatric age group.[8,9,13] Pseudocysts can occur weeks or months after the initial injury. The true incidence of pseudocyst formation after injury to the pancreas is difficult to discern because many children treated for pseudocysts at tertiary centers have been referred because of failed medical or surgical management elsewhere or because of late presentation after an unrecognized injury. While 14 (48%) of the 29 patients who presented to our facility for pancreatic trauma developed pseudocysts, only one quarter of the children seen within 24 hours of injury had this complication.

The treatment and clinical outcome of the pseudocyst cohort is demonstrated in Figure 12-3. Eight of 14 pseudocysts (57%) resolved with bowel rest and TPN (Figure 12-4). Six required further treatment because of one or more of the following situations: symptoms persisted beyond 1 month; the pseudocyst measured more than 5 centimeters in diameter and was not decreasing in size at 1 month; or the surgeon judged that spontaneous resolution of a very large pseudocyst was

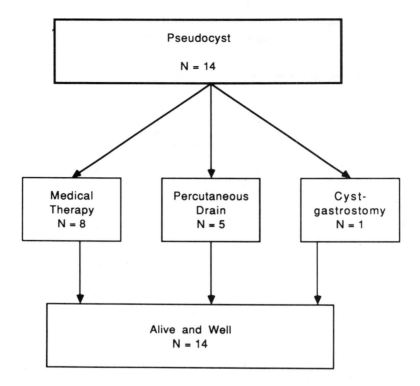

Figure 12-3. Outcome of children with pancreatic pseudocysts.

unlikely. Early in this series, 1 pseudocyst was drained operatively by cystogastrostomy. A second child, who had a "negative laparotomy" elsewhere, but developed a post-operative pseudocyst, underwent an external drainage procedure when transferred to our hospital. The pseudocyst recurred. In this patient and the subsequent 4 patients, pseudocysts were drained percutaneously aided by ultrasound or CT guidance. Table 12-2 summarizes the clinical data for these 5 patients. No child was septic at the time of pseudocyst drainage, although each child had had intermittent febrile episodes over the weeks prior to the procedure. No pseudocyst was infected at the time of drainage.

Percutaneous drainage was performed in the radiology suite with intravenous sedation and local anesthesia. In 4 cases, an 8 French pigtail catheter was introduced into the cyst after fluid had been obtained by needle puncture. In one case, a 9-centimeter pseudocyst was drained with a single puncture aspiration yielding 200 milliliters of fluid.

There were no immediate complications of percutaneous drainage. The children were allowed to eat and the catheter was removed when drainage stopped (mean 10 days). The mean hospital stay for these patients was 50 days (range 17–

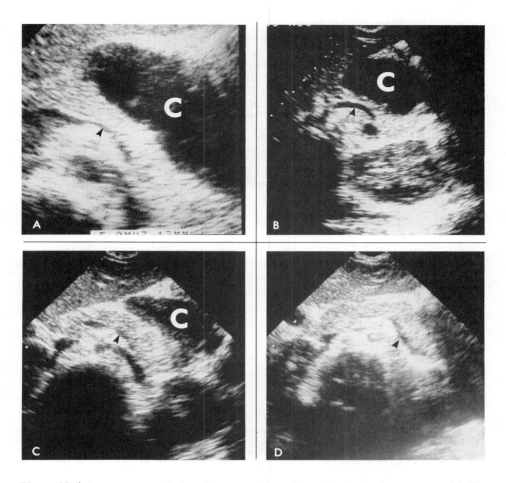

Figure 12-4. Spontaneous resolution of a pancreatic pseudocyst: Pseudocyst shown sonographically, A. 10 days, B. 24 days, and C. 34 days after trauma. D. Total resolution is noted 41 days post-injury (sv = splenic vein, c = pseudocyst).

Table 12-2. Percutaneous Pseudocyst Drainage: Patient Profile

Age (Year), Sex	Trauma to Drainage Interval	Cyst Size (ml)	Duration of Drainage	Follow-up
6, M	4 wk	12	7 day	6 yr
5, M	4 wk	15	6 day	3 yr
14, F	12 day	9	single aspiration*	1 yr
8, M	7 wk	6	15 day	9 mo
6, M	5 wk	8	10 day	7 mo

*This child underwent percutaneous drainage without catheter placement.

62 days). Serial sonograms provided accurate follow-up. No pseudocyst recurred after a mean follow-up time of 23 months (range 6 mo–6 yr).

Current Treatment Guidelines

Our current treatment protocol is noted in Table 12-3. Most children with pancreatic injuries are treated nonoperatively. Immediate operation is necessary only for those with massive abdominal bleeding, a perforated hollow viscus, and for the rare child with pancreatic transection or complex duodenopancreatic injury.

When a pancreatic injury is documented by CT and the child is hemodynamically stable, TPN is started and the bowel is left at rest. Serial ultrasound evaluation of the pancreas gives a good index of progression or regression of the pancreatic injury. Complications of pancreatic trauma are treated as they arise. Most pseudocysts that develop during treatment subside with continued medical management. Drainage is necessary for the persistent pseudocyst or for the very large cyst that appears unlikely to resolve. Percutaneous catheter drainage, which has been used only sporadically elsewhere, seems to be a safe, simple, and effective method of drainage.[13,14,15] Operative drainage procedures are reserved for those in whom percutaneous drainage fails.

The clinical syndrome of traumatic pancreatitis, which is frequently demonstrated on initial CT exam as pancreatic edema, may resolve spontaneously with bowel rest and total parenteral nutrition. The occasional case of chronic pancreati-

---

Table 12-3. Current Treatment Protocol for Pancreatic Trauma

Immediate operation

1. Pancreatic transection on CT scan: distal pancreatectomy
2. Combined pancreatoduodenal disruption: repair, duodenal decompression, drainage, and bowel rest (see text for further discussion)
3. Other injuries requiring laparotomy: intraoperative evaluation of the pancreas and treatment as necessary

All other situations

1. In-hospital observation, bowel rest, and TPN
2. Serial abdominal ultrasound and serum amylase determinations

Complications

1. Pseudocyst: percutaneous drainage if
   A. Symptomatic, persistent pseudocyst
   B. Pseudocyst 5 cm, which is not decreasing in size after one month of observation
   C. Pseudocyst thought too large to resolve spontaneously with prolonged TPN
2. Chronic pancreatitis: ERCP and distal pancreatectomy if ductal stricture present
3. Pancreatic abscess: operative debridement and drainage

tis from ductal stricture can be diagnosed using ERCP and treated with distal pancreatectomy. A pseudocyst that develops during treatment, as occurred in 48 percent of the patients in our series, usually subsides with continued medical management.

Discussion

A summary of the papers that review pancreatic trauma in children is presented in Table 12-4. Clearly, operative therapy was the mainstay of management in the past.[4-7,13] Our experience and the latest series, however, support the concept of medical management for the majority of children with traumatic lesions of the pancreas.[13] If the current protocol had been applied to all 29 children in our series, only 6 (21%) would have undergone operation, while only 2 (7%) would have required specific operative treatment for an injured pancreas.

The trend towards nonoperative treatment of pediatric abdominal injuries continues. Most splenic, hepatic, and renal injuries (which constitute the overwhelming majority of blunt abdominal trauma admissions) are now optimally treated with in-hospital observation and nonoperative supportive measures. Certain injuries still require early operative intervention. These include massive bleeding from a solid organ, hollow viscus perforation, diaphragmatic rupture, and major vascular injuries. When diagnostic studies or the physical exam dictate abdominal exploration, a deliberative search for a pancreatic lesion should be made after the major injuries are treated.

Pancreatic contusion or capsular disruption are best left alone. While some surgeons advocate suture repair of a torn pancreatic capsule,[5,9] this technique may actually convert an inconsequential injury into a more significant one. If drainage is necessary, soft atraumatic Silastic sump drains seem to be most appropriate. Many authors concur with out experience that Penrose or closed suction drains do not necessarily prevent pseudocyst formation.[16,17] A pancreatic drain should remain for a minimum of seven days to ensure drainage of a late fistula.[2,18,19]

Pancreatic injuries have been divided into four categories of increasing severity by Lucus[20] and by Smego[19] (Table 12-5). While we have not used this classification clinically, we agree that the principal determinants of prognosis in pancreatic trauma are the status of the main pancreatic duct and the integrity of the duodenum. When the duct of Wirsung is transected, distal pancreatectomy is the treatment of choice. This procedure was performed in 17 percent of the children reviewed in Table 12-5. Every attempt should be made to preserve the spleen, although Pokorny has encountered massive hemorrhage from the splenic vessels in adults when a pancreatic fistula developed following distal pancreatectomy.[5] Diabetes mellitus is unusual after pancreatic resection if even as little as 10 to 20 percent of the pancreatic parenchyma is left.[2,5] In the Parkland Hospital series,[5] only 27 percent of patients with greater than 80 percent resection required insulin and only 1 of 8 patients reported by Yellin[21] was diabetic following distal pancreatectomy with a resection line to the right of the superior mesenteric vessels. Be-

Table 12-4. Blunt Pancreatic Trauma in Children: A Review of the Literature

Author, Year	Number of Patients	Nonoperative Therapy N(%)	Operative Early N(%)	Therapy Late N(%)	Transected Pancreas N(%)	Pancreato-duodenal Injury N(%)	Death N(%)	Complications Pseudocyst N(%)	Fistula N(%)	Abscess N(%)
Grosfeld and Cooney, 1975[7]	16	0	5(31)	11(69)	1(6)	1(6)	1(6)	11(69)	0	1(6)
Meier et al, 1978[4]	16	0	16(100)		3(19)	0	3(19)	3(19)	0	0
Graham et al, 1978[5]	51*	0	47(92)*+	5(10)+	10(31)**	2(6)**	4(8)*	3(6)*	11(22)*	0
Salonen and Aarnio, 1985[6]	8	0	4(50)	4(50)	4(50)	0	0	0	0	0
Bass et al, 1988[13]	26	16(62)	10(38)		2(8)	1(4)	0	10(38)	0	0
Present Study	29	18(62)	9(31)+	3(10)+	1(3)+	0	2(7)	14(48)	0	0
Total	146	34(23)	65(63)+	23(22)+	21(14)+	4(3)+	10(7)	41(28)	11(8)	1(1)

*This report includes 10 patients (37%) with penetrating injuries and 32 patients (63%) with blunt injuries.
**Considers only children with blunt injuries
+Some children had more than one operation.

Table 12-5. Classification of Pancreatic Injury

Class 1:	Contusion, peripheral laceration, intact main ducts
Class 2:	Distal laceration, transection, or suspected duct disruption, no duodenal injury
Class 3:	Proximal laceration, transection, or suspected ductal disruption, no duodenal injury
Class 4:	Severe combined pancreatoduodenal injury

---

cause most ductal disruptions in children occur in the pancreatic body over the vertebral column, diabetes is not a likely sequela of resection. The pancreatic stump may be sewn with nonabsorbable sutures or stapled with a TA-55 3.5mm stapler.[22,23] An attempt to identify and ligate the duct with fine nonabsorbable suture should be made prior to stump closure, although it is less important if the stapler is being used.[22]

The most severe injury of this anatomic region is the combined pancreaticoduodenal disruption. Only 3 percent of children suffering blunt trauma to the pancreas had a major duodenal injury as well (see Table 12-4). Several techniques have been used to treat these difficult lesions, including simple duodenal closure with drainage, duodenal diverticularization procedures,[24] temporary gastrojejunal bypass,[25] and pancreatoduodenectomy.[26-28] The basic principles in all methods of management are as follows: closure of the duodenum; rigorous decompression of the duodenum by nasogastric tube, gastrostomy, duodenostomy, or complete gastrointestinal diversion; bowel rest and supression of pancreatic secretion, using jejunostomy feeds or TPN; and extensive drainage. Despite complex measures to repair these lesions, Feliciano reports a 30 percent mortality in an adult series of combined pancreaticoduodenal injuries with 26 percent of patients developing pancreatic fistulas, 7 percent duodenal fistulas and 17 percent intra-abdominal abscesses.[29]

Complications of pancreatic injury, especially pseudocysts, are common. Our experience and that of Bass[13] shows that over half will resolve with medical treatment alone and that persistent pseudocysts can be drained successfully using a percutaneous technique. Virtually all pancreatic fistulae close spontaneously with bowel rest and TPN. The pancreatic abscess is a rare complication that requires urgent operation. This problem carries a 100 percent mortality without operative drainage and a 30 to 50 percent mortality with drainage.[29,30] Half of the reviewed pediatric patients who developed this problem died.[7,9] Small retroperitoneal gas bubbles are pathognomonic. Operative drainage with large sump drains is mandatory. There is no place for percutaneous catheter placement because the effluent is too thick. Recently, a technique of radical debridement and open packing with regular dressing changes under anesthesia has been described,[31] resulting in a survival rate of 85 percent.

Death resulting from pancreatic injury is rare in children. While the overall death rate in the 6 pediatric series outlined was 7 percent, no child died from complications of the pancreatic injury. In a 1972 series of 30 pediatric patients,

Stone[9] reported 2 deaths related to pancreatic trauma, one from pancreatic abscess and the other from complications of a duodenal fistula in a combined pancreatoduodenal injury. We chose to exclude this series from Table 12-4 because it was not possible to separate the penetrating injuries (which constituted 67% of the experience) from the blunt injuries.

Many authors assert that early operative therapy will decrease the morbidity of pancreatic injury.[1,2,16,17] Our recent experience demonstrates an excellent overall outcome in children managed initially with careful observation, TPN, and bowel rest. The incidence of post-traumatic pseudocyst may possibly be greater with this conservative approach, but the efficacy and simplicity of percutaneous drainage minimizes the consequences.

Summary

Pancreatic trauma in children almost always results from blunt trauma to the epigastrium. The diagnosis is frequently delayed because the initial signs and symptoms may be mild. Serum amylase is a good screening test, but CT scan is the diagnostic study of choice. Operative therapy is no longer indicated for all children who present with pancreatic injuries. An initial course of TPN and bowel rest is appropriate, except when a transected pancreas combined pancreatoduodenal injury or other major intra-abdominal trauma requires laparotomy. Three-quarters of children who start with conservative management will never need any further therapy. Serial ultrasound examination is the best way to follow these patients until symptoms resolve. Late complications of pancreatic trauma, including pancreatitis, fistula, abscess, and pseudocyst, occur even following optimal management of the acute injury. Most of these problems will resolve spontaneously with medical treatment, although prolonged hospitalization is not uncommon. Pseudocysts have been treated effectively by percutaneous catheter drainage. Successful outcome in pancreatic trauma requires prompt recognition and treatment of both the acute problem and the late complications.

References

1. Nance FC: Management of injuries to the stomach, duodenum and pancreas. In Worth MH Jr (ed): Principles and Practice of Trauma Care. Baltimore, Williams and Wilkins, 1982
2. Jones RC: Management of pancreatic trauma. Am J Surg, 150:698, 1985
3. Stone HH, Fabian TC, Satiani B, Turkleson M: Experiences in the management of pancreatic trauma. J Trauma 21:257, 1981
4. Meier D, Gravier L, Votteler T, Coln D: Blunt trauma to the pancreas in children. South Med J 71:895, 1978
5. Graham JM, Pokorny WJ, Mattox K, Jordon G: Surgical management of acute pancreatic injuries in children. J Pediatr Surg 13:178, 1978
6. Salonen IS, Aarnio P: Treatment of acute pancreatic injuries in childhood. Ann Chir Gynaecol 74:167, 1985

7. Grosfeld JL, Cooney DR: Pancreatic and gastrointestinal trauma in children. Pediatr Clin North Am 22:365, 1975
8. Gorenstein A, O'Halpin D, Wesson D et al: Blunt injury to the pancreas in children: Selective management based on ultrasound. J Pediatr Surg 22:1110, 1987
9. Stone HH: Pancreatic and duodenal trauma in children. J Pediatr Surg 7:670, 1972
10. Pearl R, Wesson D, Spence L et al: Splenic injury: A 5-year update with improved results and changing criteria for conservative management. J Pediatr Surg 24:121, 1989
11. Giacomantonio M, Filler RM, Rich RH: Blunt hepatic trauma in children: Experience with operative and non-operative management. J Pediatr Surg 19:519, 1984
12. Jeffrey RB, Federle MP, Crass RA: Computed tomography in pancreatic trauma. Radiology 147:491, 1983
13. Bass J, Dilorenz M, Desjardins M et al: Blunt pancreatic injury in children—the role of percutaneous external drainage in the treatment of pancreatic pseudocysts. J Pediatr Surg 23:721, 1988
14. Windle R, Finlay D, Neoptolemos JP: Needle aspiration in the treatment of pancreatic pseudocyst in childhood. Ann R Coll Surg Engl 65:331, 1983
15. Arata JA, Jaffe ME, Matlak ME: Percutaneous drainage of traumatic pancreatic pseudocysts in childhood. Am J Radiol 152:591, 1989
16. Jones RC: JL: Changing trends in the management of pancreatic trauma. (in discussion of Cogbill TH, Moore EE, and Kashuk JL) Arch Surg 117:722, 1982
17. Weigelt JA (ed): Trauma Overview. Selected Readings in General Surgery 14:1, 1987
18. Jones RC: Management of pancreatic trauma. Ann Surg 187:555, 1978
19. Smego DR, Richardson JD, Flint L: Determinants of outcome in pancreatic trauma. J Trauma 25:771, 1985
20. Lucas CE: Diagnosis and treatment of pancreatic and duodenal injury. Surg Clin North Am 57:49, 1977
21. Yellin AE, Vecchione TR, Donovan AJ: Distal pancreatectomy for pancreatic trauma. Am J Surg 124:135, 1972
22. Anderson DK, Bolman RM III, Moylan JA JR: Management of penetrating pancreatic injuries: Subtotal pancreatectomy using the autosuture stapler. J Trauma 120:347, 1980
23. Fitzgibbons TJ, Yellin AE, Maruyama M, Donovan A: Management of the transected pancreas following distal pancreatectomy. Surg Gynecol Obstet 154:225, 1982
24. Berne CJ, Donovan AJ, White E: Duodenal diverticulization for duodenal and pancreatic injury. Am J Surg 127:503, 1974
25. Vaughan GD, Frazier OH, Graham D et al: The use of pyloric exclusion in the management of severe duodenal injuries. Am J Surg 134:785, 1977
26. Lowe RF, Saletta JD, Moss GS: Pancreaticoduodenectomy for penetrating pancreatic trauma. J Trauma 17:732, 1977
27. Oreskovich MR, Carrico CJ: Pancreaticoduodenectomy for trauma: A viable option? Am J Surg 147:618, 1984
28. Thal AP, Wilson RF: A pattern of severe blunt trauma to the region of the pancreas. Surg Gynecol Obstet, 119:73, 1964
29. Feliciano DV, Martin TM, Cruise P et al: Management of combined pancreaticoduodenal injuries. Ann Surg 205:673, 1987
30. Owens BJ III, Hamit HF: Pancreatic abscess and pseudocyst. Arch Surg 112:42, 1977
31. Bradley El III, Fulenwider JT: Open treatment of pancreatic abscess. Surg Gynecol Obstet 159:509, 1984

CHAPTER 13

Extracorporeal Life Support in Pediatric Trauma

Robert H. Bartlett and Harry L. Anderson III

T he technique of venoarterial extracorporeal circulation (cardiopulmonary by-pass) is familiar to all surgeons who have had experience in a cardiac surgery service during their training. During cardiac surgery, venous blood is drained from the right atrium and vena cavae to the heart/lung machine, where oxygen is added, CO_2 removed, the temperature controlled, and the arterialized blood is perfused into the aorta. The development of this technique by Gibbon made cardiac surgery possible. For the last 20 years, many surgical investigators have studied the physiology of extracorporeal circulation, and modified the heart/lung machine to permit its use for days or weeks rather than a few hours in the operating room.[1] This technique has been used primarily for hypoxic patients with respiratory failure, and it uses a membrane lung. Hence, it has been described as *extracorporeal membrane oxygenation* (ECMO). However, this term is incomplete and a better description is *extracorporeal life support* (ECLS). Although initial anecdotal reports were encouraging, a 1978 multi-center randomized study found that only 10 percent of adult patients with respiratory failure who were treated with ECLS survived.[2] Recently, several groups from Europe and Canada have reported 50 percent survival in adult respiratory failure, and there is a resurgence of interest in this technique in adult intensive care units (ICUs).[3,4] However, the most successful application has been in newborn infants with respiratory failure.[5]

The first clinical trials of extracorporeal support in neonatal respiratory failure showed that extracorporeal circulation could be conducted in newborn infants, although all of the infants died of their primary disease.[6-8] In 1975, our research group reported the first successful use of extracorporeal circulation for newborn respiratory failure.[9] By 1980, we had studied 40 cases with 22 survivors at the University of California, Irvine.[10] Between 1980 and 1989, we treated 177 cases at the University of Michigan with 164 survivors. Most of these children are healthy in follow-up, and our ECLS technique has become quite standardized. Many other neonatal centers have learned the techniques of extracorporeal circulation and

Supported in part by a grant from the National Institutes of Health.

ECMO is now established as standard management for term and near-term infants who fail to respond to conventional ventilator therapy.

Following the success in neonatal and adult respiratory failure, attention turned to the application of ECLS to pediatrics. Lethal respiratory failure is unusual in children. When it occurs, it is usually the result of viral pneumonia, bacterial pneumonia, congenital disease of the lung, pulmonary capillary leakage secondary to distant infection or ischemic tissue, or accidental injury. Although few cases of its use have been reported, the future of ECLS for children who sustain lung injury looks promising. This chapter describes the potential applications of ECLS systems in pediatric trauma.

Patient Selection

Drowning leads the list of accidental lung injury in children, followed by smoke inhalation, chemical aspiration, direct pulmonary contusion, and pulmonary capillary injury (ARDS) following extrathoracic traumatic injury. Extracorporeal life support has been used for each of these applications.[11-16] The indication for ECLS is acute severe cardiac or pulmonary failure that is potentially reversible within one or two weeks of time, during which ECLS can be carried out with few complications. While this definition is easy to describe in adjectives, it is much more difficult in nouns. Obviously, ECLS is invasive and has inherent risks, so it should be used only when conventional treatment is failing and the prognosis is poor. Criteria for defining this situation exists for adults[2,17] and neonates,[1] but not for children. Currently, a major study is underway to determine the epidemiology, risk factors, and quantitative mortality risk in pediatric respiratory failure.

Until data are available for children, we have used the criteria that apply to adult patients with acute respiratory failure—transpulmonary shunt greater than 30 percent and static compliance less than 0.5 cc/cmH$_2$O despite optimal pharmacologic and ventilator management. Another indication is barotrauma. Some children may have extensive air leaks that preclude ventilation although oxygenation is adequate.

Contraindications include conditions incompatible with normal life after lung recovery (such as major brain injury), congenital or acquired immunodeficiency states, and mechanical ventilation for more than 5 to 10 days (as an indication of irreversible ventilator-induced lung injury). Relative contraindications include actual or potential bleeding conditions that may be exacerbated by heparinization (such as recent head injury or recent major operation).

The ECLS Circuit and Management of Extracorporeal Circulation

The circuit includes a servo-regulated roller pump, membrane lung, heat exchanger, and polyvinylchloride tubing and connectors (Figure 12-1). Blood is drained by means of a cannula in the right internal jugular or femoral vein by a

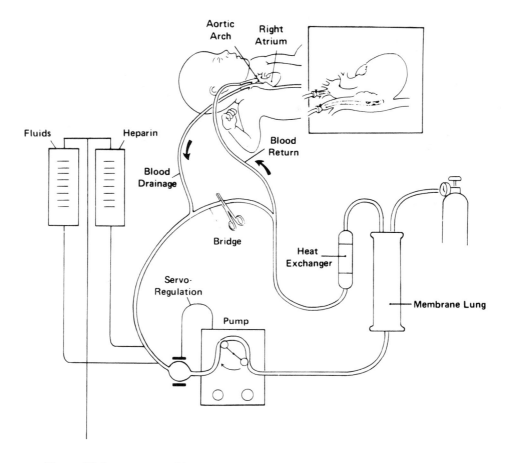

Figure 13-1. Extracorporeal life support circuit diagram in a typical neonatal application.

gravity siphon (100 cm) to a small distensible bladder. The bladder and a "bladder box" microswitch act as a servoregulator of the roller pump. The pump is turned off whenever the pump flow exceeds the venous blood return. In addition, this system avoids air embolism by turning off the pump if a large air bubble is entrained in the venous line.

Blood passes through an occlusive roller pump and is perfused through a silicone rubber membrane Kolobow Sci-Med® lung. The size of the artificial lung is selected to provide complete cardiopulmonary support. A given artificial lung has a "rated flow," which specifies the maximum blood flow rate at which normal venous blood perfusate leaves the oxygenator 95 percent saturated. Therefore, the artificial lung chosen for a given case must have a rated flow equivalent to or greater than the cardiac output of the patient.

heparin. This will minimize much of the bleeding complications, although thrombocytopenia will still be present to some extent and will require treatment.

The heparin-coated life support system will have a major application in pediatric trauma care, particularly in burn and smoke inhalation injury and in direct tissue injury cases, in which extracorporeal support is rarely used now because of the risk of bleeding. With the advent of heparin-coated systems and simple percutaneous venovenous cannulation vascular access, the threshold to use extracorporeal support will be much lower. Extracorporeal life support will be used for children with 30 percent mortality risk rather than the current 90 percent mortality risk indications. We hope this will result in less ventilator-induced lung injury and better rates of survival in these patients.

Summary

Extracorporeal life support has been used occasionally for children with accidental injury. The best results have been in drowning and chemical aspiration injuries. ECLS should be considered in any child with major respiratory failure. When it is used, it should be instituted before ventilator-induced lung injury has occurred, typically within a few days of the time of intubation.

References

1. Hirschl RB, Bartlett RH: Extracorporeal membrane oxygenation (ECMO) support in cardiorespiratory failure. In Tompkins R (ed): Advances in Surgery, p 189–211. Chicago, Year Book Medical Publishers, 1987
2. Zapol WM, Snider MT, Hill JD et al: Extracorporeal membrane oxygenation in severe acute respiratory failure: A randomized prospective study. JAMA 179:2193–2196, 1979
3. Gattinoni L, Pesenti A, Mascheroni D et al: Low-frequency positive-pressure ventilation with extracorporeal CO_2 removal in severe acute respiratory failure. JAMA 256:881–886, 1986
4. Pesenti A, Kolobow T, Gattinoni L: Extracorporeal respiratory support in the adult. Trans ASAIO 34:1006–1008, 1988
5. Toomasian JM, Snedecor SM, Cornell RG et al: National experience with extracorporeal membrane oxygenation for newborn respiratory failure: Data from 715 cases. Trans ASAIO 11:140–147. 1988
6. Rashkind WJK, Freeman A, Klein D et al: Evaluation of a disposable plastic, low-volume, pumpless oxygenator as a lung substitute. J Pediatr 66:94, 1965
7 Dorson WJ, Baker E, Cohen ML et al: A perfusion system for infants. Trans Am Soc Artif Intern Organs 15:155, 1969
8. White JJ, Andrews HG, Reisemberg H et al: Prolonged respiratory support in newborn infants with a membrane oxygenator. Surgery 70:288, 1971
9. Bartlett RH, Gazzaniga AB: Extracorporeal circulation for cardiopulmonary failure. Current Problems in Surgery, vol 15. Chicago, Year Book Medical Publishers, 1978
10. Bartlett RH, Andrews AF, Toomasian JM et al: Extracorporeal membrane oxygenation for newborn respiratory failure: 45 cases. Surgery 92:425, 1982

11. Snider MT, Campbell DB, Kofke WA et al: Venovenous perfusion of adults and children with severe acute respiratory distress syndrome. Trans ASAIO 34:1014–1020, 1988

12. Klein MD, Arensman RM, Weber TR et al: Pediatric ECMO: Directions for new developments. Trans ASAIO 34:978–985, 1988

13. Ortiz RM, Cilley RE, Bartlett RH: Extracorporeal membrane oxygenation in pediatric respiratory failure. Pediatr Clin North Am 34:39–46, 1987

14. Redmond CR, Graves ED, Falterman KW et al: Extracorporeal membrane oxygenation for respiratory and cardiac failure in infants and children. J Thorac Cardiovasc Surg 93:199–204, 1987

15. Anderson HL, Attori RJ, Custer JR et al: Extracorporeal membrane oxygenation (ECMO) for pediatric cardiopulmonary failure. J Thorac Cardiovasc Surg (in press)

16. Durandy Y, Batisse A, Chevalier JY: A new extracorporeal assist device = Initial clinical experience in pediatric patients. Intensive Care Med (abstract) 14(supp 1):268, 1988

17. Bartlett RH, Morris AH, Fairley HB et al: A prospective study of acute hypoxic respiratory failure. Chest 89 5:684–689, 1986.

18. Klein MD, Andrews AF, Wesley JR et al: Venovenous perfusion in ECMO for newborn respiratory insufficiency: A clinical comparison with venoarterial perfusion. Ann Surg 201:520–526, 1985

19. Zwischenberger JB, Cilley RE, Kirsh MM et al: Does continuous monitoring of mixed venous oxygen saturation (SvO_2) accurately reflect oxygen delivery (DO_2) and oxygen consumption (VO_2) following coronary artery bypass grafting (CABG)? Surg Forum 37:66–68, 1986

20. Anderson HL, Cilley RE, Zwischenberger JB, Bartlett RH: Thrombocytopenia in neonates after extracorporeal membrane oxygenation. Trans ASAIO 32:534–537, 1986

21. Heiss KF, Pettit B, Hirschl RB et al: Renal insufficiency and volume overload in neonatal ECMO managed by continuous ultrafiltration. Trans ASAIO 33:557–560, 1987

22. Toomasian JM, Hsu L-C, Hirschl RB et al: Evaluation of Duraflo II heparin coating in prolonged extracorporeal membrane oxygenation. Trans ASAIO 34:410–414, 1988

23. Mottaghy K, Oedekoven B, Poppel K et al: Heparin-free long term extracorporeal circulation using bioactive surfaces. Trans ASAIO (in press)

CHAPTER 14

Infections and Antibiotics

Thomas C. Shope

L ittle has been written specifically about trauma, infections, and the use of antibiotics in pediatric patients. Some argue that organisms introduced during
trauma in children are not essentially different than those in adult trauma, and that
subsequent management of infections should follow from lessons learned in adult
studies. However, I believe there are important differences between pediatric and
adult populations, differences that have an impact on management decisions.

The first is obvious: pediatric patients are not little adults, but are developing
human beings, and, with respect to infectious diseases, children are colonized by
microflora that changes with age. For example, during the first two years of life,
cultures of the colon regularly yield *Clostridium difficile*—an organism rare among
adults. The occurrence of group A β-*hemolytic streptococcus* in the nasopharynx
under age two is quite rare, and first-time colonization with *Haemophilus influenzae* type b or pneumococci in a previously inexperienced child carries risk of
pathogenic invasion and secondary disease. Thus, when trauma has occurred in a
child, the initial assessment of risk of infection must take into account the patient's
age. A second aspect of age is related to the pharmacology of certain antibiotics.
The quinolines, a large new class of antibiotics, are not approved for use in children because of their deleterious effect on growing long bones and joints. Another
example is the vast difference in the elimination constants observed during the
first few weeks of life for drugs like the penicillins and the aminoglycosides. In
newborns, calculations of drug dose need to take into account altered renal excretion. By the same token, the usual sensitivity patterns and predictions of microbial
susceptibility are based on expected concentration of a drug in an adult. Sensitivity
predictions must be interpreted with caution in a child, whose renal function, hepatic function, intestinal absorption, and body size may vary simply because the
child is growing.

Recognizing that age is the major consideration that separates the pediatric
and adult populations, what principles are involved in the initial decision making
concerning treatment of potential or real infections present with pediatric trauma?
Recognition of infection is straightforward. The usual signs and symptoms of infection are reliably present in pediatric patients just as in older patients. Thus, fever,
local signs of inflammation, an elevated white blood cell count with predominant

polymorphonuclear leukocytes, and an elevated sedimentation rate are all reliable factors that suggest infection. Once infection is recognized, a suitable antimicrobial must be chosen. A much broader armamentarium is available for the management of bacterial infections than fungal, parasitic, or viral infections. Yet, there are antimicrobials in place for the latter three groups of infectious microorganisms. A reasonable approach is for the physician to select antimicrobials that are effective over a broad range of microorganisms, while simultaneously obtaining cultures and gram stains to better define the infecting organism(s). Once the infectious organism has been identified, therapy should be tapered to a specific, appropriate antibiotic. Selection of the initial antibiotic should be guided by the ease of use. Serum levels should be available if the drug is toxic, or a less toxic alternative should be selected. The drug chosen should diffuse to the infected site and potentially infected sites. If therapy will be prolonged, consideration should be given to the potential for oral administration of the same or a related antibiotic.

Any discussion of antibiotics related to trauma must consider the issue of prophylactic use during the immediate post-trauma period. Use of prophylactic antibiotics should be short-term, at a relatively low cost, and with the goal of broad coverage. Consideration must given to whether the wound is dirty or clean, its location, and if generation of the wound interfered with the integrity of normally sterile spaces, or passed through a normally colonized space into a normally sterile space. It has been recognized that it is impossible to prevent bacterial overgrowth when managing a wound that is contiguous with the outside surface. Initially, all one can hope to accomplish is to retard the replication of microorganisms at the site long enough to allow the patient to mount an effective immune response. If this cannot happen within 48 to 96 hours, then organisms that survived the initial use of broad spectrum antibiotics will emerge and begin to dominate the flora of the affected site. Eventually, if the initial antibiotic coverage was broad enough, the organisms that emerge as dominant will be those organisms that are highly resistant to broad-spectrum antibiotics. The most common trauma in which overgrowth occurs is burns of large body surfaces. However, there are many other examples, such as repeated bladder irrigation, intubation with an endotracheal tube, and paranasal sinus infections secondary to nasogastric tubes.

The principles of appropriate selection of antibiotics and initial management of traumatic wounds can be given in a relatively simple set of guidelines. First, the physican should know the kind of organism that is likely to be present, or make a reasonable guess based on the clinical information available. Second, make an accurate assessment of the antibiotic susceptibility patterns prevalent in your community. If, for instance, you never see multiply resistant *Staphylococcus aureus,* then there may never be a good rationale for using a drug like vancomycin in initial care of a traumatic wound. Finally, consider the appropriate host factors, such as the patient's age, previous treatment with broad-spectrum antibiotics, and specific age-related characteristics that have to do with the pharmacokinetics and pharmacology of the antibiotics that you wish to use. Holding these principles and guidelines in mind, the discussion below will address issues specific to various foci of trauma.

Bites and Other Skin Wounds

Human and animal bites are relatively common sources of trauma to the head, neck, and extremities. While these bites may appear innocuous initially, they do serve as an important source of subsequent infections. Studies that have used techniques adequate to detect anaerobes indicate that indigenous oral flora colonize wounds more often than common skin flora.[1,2] The most prevalent facultative organisms include streptococci, *Eikenella corrodens,* and *S. aureus.* The most common anaerobes isolated include *Bacteroides, Peptococcus,* and *Peptostreptococcus.* In addition to the above-named organisms, animal bites (particularly cat and dog) may be associated with *Pasteurella multocida.* The organisms of both human and animal oral cavities are uniquely susceptible to penicillin. In fact, *E. corrodens* is susceptible to penicillin and ampicillin, but resistant to the penicillinase-resistant drugs such as oxacillin, methacillin, nafcillin, and clindamycin. Thus, penicillin remains the antibiotic of choice as initial therapy.

Spider bites may require management of the effects of the toxins injected, but are rarely infected as a primary event and require no initial antibiotic coverage. However, manipulation of the bite site during surgical management of the local reaction may result in the subsequent requirement for antibiotic intervention. The antibiotics chosen should be effective against the skin flora normally associated with incisional wounds.

Bites from venomous snakes may be associated with extensive tissue destruction and devitalization that predisposes to infection from the snake's normal oral flora. The presence of fecal flora is more common secondary to snake bites than in animal or human bites, presumably because as the snake ingests live prey, the prey defecates in the snake's mouth.[3] Thus, organisms such as *Pseudomonas aeroginosa, proteus* species, coagulase-negative staphylococci, and *clostridium* species, as well as *Bacteroides fragilis* and *Arizona hinshawii* may be present in the bites from venomous snakes. Although not well worked out, antimicrobials chosen specifically to cover potential gram-negative enteric organisms should be included in the initial regimen until cultures are returned from the laboratory and the flora can be better defined.

Not all bites become infected. The effect that immediate first aid has on the bacteriology of wounds or subsequent infection rates is not known. Most people who have been bitten will attempt self-therapy by washing the wounds with soap and water or using hydrogen peroxide or topical salves. Estimates vary, but up to 30 percent of "self-treated" wounds subsequently develop infection.[4,5] Patients who seek medical care 24 to 48 hours after sustaining a bite wound almost always present with established infection.

Management of animal bites includes an initial thorough cleansing with copious amounts of sterile solution, accompanied by appropriate debridement and trimming of devitalized skin flaps and, if anatomy permits, probing of deep penetrating wounds. The decision of whether to close the wound primarily after cleansing and debridement remains controversial, but observations that even well managed wounds (including those treated with antimicrobials) carry a 20 percent infection risk seem to mediate against primary closure unless absolutely necessary. Penicillin or ampicillin is the most active agent against *P. multocida* and other oral aerobic and anaerobic bacteria of dogs and cats. Tetracycline is a good alternative for penicillin-allergic patients although it should not be administered to pregnant women or children. Erythromycin is an effective alternative against approximately 50 percent of *P. multocida* organisms. Clindamycin and penicillinase-resistant penicillins and cephalosporins are inappropriate because they are not generally effective against *P. multocida* and *E. corrodens*. Finally, if *S. aureus* is suspected, a combination of penicillin and a penicillinase-resistant pencillin should be used. Antibiotic treatment for 5 days appears to be adequate for wounds that are treated early; duration of treatment may exceed 7 to 14 days for those that present with established infections.

Wound Infections

The usual wound infection that occurs 2 to 3 days after initial wound management is almost always associated with skin flora, predominantly *S. aureus* and β-*hemolytic streptococcus*. These wounds can be appropriately cultured and are usually very efficiently managed with nafcillin or dicloxacillin

Two related issues must be considered in the initial management of bites and other skin wounds: when should tetanus precautions be considered, and when should rabies control measures be instituted?

Care of Persons Exposed to Tetanus or with Tetanus-Prone Injuries

Individuals who have completed a series of 4 tetanus toxoid injections at any time in their lives are at extremely low risk of developing tetanus. After primary immunization with tetanus toxoid, anti-toxin antibodies persist at protective levels in most persons for at least 10 years; and the ability to react promptly to a booster injection persists for an even longer time. Thus, for previously tetanus-immunized individuals with clean, non-tetanus-prone wounds, no immunization is necessary unless the patient has not had a booster in the previous decade. If the patient has not had a booster injection, one should be given, not because of the threat of tetanus, but because it is good preventive medicine management. For tetanus-prone wounds in a previously immunized patient, treatment is required if the last complete series dose was fewer than 5 years prior to the injury. If the last dose was more than 5 years ago, adult tetanus-diphtheria toxoid (Td) is given. Passive protection with tetanus immune globulin is not indicated for patients with clean, minor wounds regardless of their immunization status, or for tetanus-prone wounds if there have been 3 or more previous injections of tetanus toxoid. However, patients with more serious wounds, who have had fewer than 3 previous injections of tetanus toxoid, should receive intramuscular tetanus-immune globulin, human, at a dose of 500 to 3000 U. The optimum therpeutic dose has not been established. Efforts should be made to initiate completion of immunization in individuals who do not have complete immunization at the time their tetanus-prone wound occurred. There is no role for prophylactic antibiotic administration to control the possibility of tetanus in a tetanus-prone wound.

Rabies Control Measures

The decision to use rabies control measures involves accurate assessment of the risk that the patient has been exposed to rabies. Exposure to rabies results from a break in the skin caused by the teeth or claws of a rabid animal or by the contamination of scratches, abrasions, or mucus membranes with saliva from a rabid animal. Local health departments routinely monitor local animal species for the presence of rabies. The estimate for risk of exposure, therefore, relates to where the animal was at the time of exposure; whether the bite was provoked; if the animal was wild or domesticated; and, if domesticated, whether it was immunized. In the United States, skunks, raccoons, and bats are more likely to be infected than other animals, but foxes, coyotes, cattle, dogs, and cats occasionally are infected. Bites of squirrels, rats, or rabbits rarely require specific anti-rabies prohylaxis.

Treatment includes appropriate care of the local wound, which should be thoroughly flushed and cleaned with soap and water. If immunoprophylaxis is to be used, optimal therapy requires both passive and active immunoprophylaxis. Active immunization should use human diploid cell vaccine (1 ml) given intramuscularly on the first day of treatment, and repeated on days 3, 7, 14, and 28 after the first dose. Testing of sera after immunization with human diploid cell vaccine generally is not necessary because 5 doses reliably give protective antibody responses. Passive immunization using human rabies immune globulin should be used concommitant with the first dose of vaccine for post-exposure prophylaxis. The recommended dose is 20 IU of human rabies immune globulin/kg of body weight. Approximately one half of the antibody preparation is used to infiltrate the wound; the remainder is given intramuscularly.

Head Injury

Penetrating injury to the head disrupts the barriers that normally separate colonized cavities and sterile structures. Both the aerobic and anaerobic bacteria that form the flora of the upper airways have limited invasive properties, unless associated conditions permit their movement into deeper, normally sterile structures. In this case, the major anaerobic pathogens in head and neck infections are *Fusobacter nucleatum, Bacteroides melaninogenicus,* and the anaerobic gram-positive cocci.[6] Fusobacteria are harbored in the normal flora of the oropharynx, saliva, and gingival crevices. *B. melaninogenicus* and anaerobic spirochetes are concentrated in the gingival crevice in persons past the age of puberty. Anaerobic cocci are widely distributed in the upper airways, accounting for approximately 15 percent of all bacteria in saliva. Aerobes colonizing these same spaces are predominantly *Streptococcus pneumoniae* and non-typable *H. influenzae* organisms. To a much lesser extent, *Branhamella catarrhalis,* and occasionally *S. aureus* and both α-rhemolytic streptococci and β-hemolytic streptococci may be involved. Both *H. influenzae* and *B. catarrhalis* organisms may produce β-lactamases that render simple β-lactam molecules ineffective. Thus, a β-lactam-resistant cephalosporin (such as cefamandole or cefazolin) is a good initial choice to manage contaminated penetrating head wounds until the microorganisms involved can be more specifically identified. However, if there has been penetration into the cranial vault or a CSF communication, neither of these first-generation cephalosporins will penetrate the blood–brain barrier effectively, as discussed below.

Trauma to the head may result in communication of the subarachnoid space with the paranasal sinuses, nasopharynx, or middle ear. Meningitis can result from such communications, days or even years after the trauma has occurred. Communications with the paranasal sinuses, nasopharynx, and the middle ear usually result from fractures of the paranasal sinuses, cribriform plate, or petrous bone, respectively. In over 80 percent of infections of the subarachnoid space associated with skull fractures, the causative agent is *S. pneumoniae.*[7] However, if the patient has received antimicrobial prophylaxis (especially with penicillin or ampicillin), gram-negative bacilli are more likely to be the causative organisms. Controversy exists over the value of prophylactic antimicrobial use to prevent meningitis in the presence of spinal fluid leaks. Most studies indicate that prophylactic antibiotic use will prevent invasion by antibiotic-suseptible organisms, but will not prevent eventual invasion and subsequent space infection. Therefore, management of bacterial infections secondary to spinal fluid leakage requires a cephalosporin that effectively penetrates spinal fluid. Examples include third-generation cephalosporins such as ceftriaxone and cefotaxime. An equally effective alternative is the choice of a combination of ampicillin and chloramphenicol.

Pulmonary Problems

The contents of the chest are normally sterile; management of penetrating wounds would relate to the potential for contamination caused by the nature of the trauma, and the likelihood that skin contaminants might be involved in infection of the wound. Blunt trauma to the chest wall, such as might result in pulmonary contusions, should not require any antibiotic intervention.

A number of potential infectious pulmonary problems can follow severe burns. Smoke inhalation may be associated with prominent damage that most frequently would become apparent 2 to 3 days post-injury. Pulmonary problems may arise from thermal damage to the chest wall with a resulting decrease in compliance to the chest wall and, therefore, incomplete respiratory effort. In addition, post-injury hyperventilation and subsequent decrease in tidal volume may lead to atelectasis and pneumonia. Severely burned individuals may have a high requirement for nutrition, necessitating large-volume nasogastric tube feedings with the distinct possibility for overload aspiration associated with too rapid fluid administration. Finally, diminished mucociliary function from destruction of airway epithelium may lead to obstruction and infection from direct damage. Use of inhaled antibiotics or steroid sprays to prevent bacterial superinfections following smoke inhalation have been uniformly unsuccessful and play no role in the initial management of patients with smoke inhalation.[8] If treatment is to be undertaken, it must be specific for the organism(s) involved. Pneumonia secondary to severe burns is as likely to occur from hematogenous spread of organisms from the wound surface or an infected venous site as it is from aspiration of oropharyngeal microorganisms.[9] Thus, following thermal or smoke inhalation injury, every effort must be made to specifically identify the organisms involved in the pulmonary infiltrate.

Finally, a very common question occurs in treatment of the patient who, for whatever reason, has been intubated and is on respiratory ventilator assistance. Endotracheal tubes invariably become colonized by organisms in the oropharynx, and growth is enhanced by the moist environment associated with mechanical ventilators. Surveillance cultures rapidly reveal the presence of organisms such as *Pseudomonas, Klebsiella, Enterobacter, Serratia,* and *Citrobacter,* as well as a wide array of gram-positive organisms such as streptococci. Such patients frequently present with elevated body temperature, but no focus of infection, leading to the question of how to interpret the significance of organisms being recovered from the endotracheal tube cultures. Unless there is demonstrated change in the pulmonary infiltrate in lung volume and respiratory rate, or increased pulmonary resistance, there is very little rationale for reacting to the presence of organisms in the endotracheal equipment. In this respect, periodic cultures (every 2–3 days) may be of some surveillance value in case the patient's symptomatology indicates that one or another of the organisms has become invasive, but the presence alone of microflora does not require antibiotic administration. This is another good example of the principle that antibiotics given in a preventive effort over a prolonged period of time ultimately fail to prevent secondary infections, which are always with organisms resistant to the initial antibiotics.

Abdomen

Traumatic injury to the abdomen may penetrate the viscera, leading to enteric spillage, splenic rupture, and pancreatic or hepatic injury. Our discussion will focus first on penetrating injury of the gastrointestinal tract involving enteric spillage. The mucus membranes of the stomach, upper small bowel, lower small bowel, large bowel, and vagina each have a microflora specific to the location. Normally, the mucosal factors, including the mucus membrane itself, and acid or alkaline secretions, control the invasive potential of the microflora colonizing the membrane. However, disruption of the mucus membrane allows for introduction of pathogens into areas that, when colonized, become ideal environments for the replication and subsequent damage by microorganisms. The stomach in its fasting state is normally nearly sterile. The few organisms found there are generally facultative, gram-positive salivary microorganisms such as *Lactobacillus* and various kinds of streptococci. During or immediately after a meal, the microbial content of the stomach increases for several hours. Likewise, the upper small bowel microflora is sparse ($<10^3$ cfu/ml) and the microflora are similar to those found in the stomach. However in the ileum, *E. coli* and *enterococci* and obligate anaerobes such as *B. fragilis* are found in considerable concentration. Only in the colon are massive amounts of bacteria commonly encountered ($>10^{11}$ bacteria/ml of feces); the content of the colon is practically pure bacteria. Obligate anaerobes such as *B. fragilis,* and *Bifidobacterium* species outnumber *E. coli* by approximately 1000:1. Other bacteria found in lesser quantities include viridans streptococci, *Enterococci, Eubacterium* species, and *Clostridium perfringens.* There are small variations in the microflora in various locations in the bowel related to age, but these variations are minor and do not have an impact on the dominant species of any particular region of the gastrointestinal tract.

There is little information about organisms colonizing vaginal mucosa prior to adolescence. Quantitative studies in sexually active women during the child-bearing period have revealed that the predominant vaginal microflora is composed of five to seven species, and that anaerobes are approximately ten times more numerous than facultative organisms. The most frequent isolates are obligate or facultative anaerobic *Lactobacilli,* non-enterococcal streptococci, anaerobic gram positive cocci, and *Bacteroidaceae* other than *B. fragilis.* When specifically looked for, *Gardnerella vaginalis* and *Haemophilus vaginalis* in high counts have been found to be slightly less frequent than *Lactobacilli* in the vaginal secretions of normal women. On the other hand, colonic organisms, such as *B. fragilis, Enterobacteriaceae,* and *Enterococci* are rarely found as predominant components of the normal vaginal flora, and probably proliferate in this site only under exceptional circumstances. However, the bacteriologic characteristics of intra-abdominal infection following female genital tract trauma is quite similar to the peritonitis that occurs secondary to enteric spillage. Anaerobes such as *Bacteroides* and anaerobic gram-positive cocci are found in the majority of infections, along with *E. coli* and *Streptococci,* and infections are usually mixed.

Factors favoring the proliferation of organisms within the peritoneal cavity are at present incompletely understood. However, damage caused by *p*H changes secondary to acidity or alkalinity, as well as damage caused by bile or pancreatic secretions, stimulate an outpouring of serum protein and electrolytes from the blood into the peritoneal cavity. Widespread necrosis may result from enzymatic digestion. Taken together, the subsequent damage creates very appropriate conditions for the replication of both aerobic and anaerobic bacteria. Most significantly, free hemoglobin enhances peritoneal infection through mechanisms not well understood at present, but which may relate to the presence of free iron. Iron is required for bacterial metabolism, and free iron may greatly enhance infections because of certain microorganisms such as *Enterobacteriaceae* and *C. perfringens*. In addition, experimental evidence demonstrates that intraperitoneal hemoglobin depresses the influx of granulocytes into the peritoneal cavity.[10] Proliferation of microflora in the peritoneal cavity not only causes a widespread peritonitis, but eventually leads to pockets of inflammatory foci that develop into multiple abscesses. In addition to the local proliferation and damage caused by microflora, endotoxin is commonly elaborated by gram-negative organisms, both facultative as well as anaerobic. The absorption of endotoxin into the circulatory system leads to widespread systemic impact.

Finally, many intra-abdominal infections appear to be synergistic. Although it is probable that the majority of bacteria isolated in mixed infections are nonpathogenic by themselves, their presence may be essential, nevertheless, for the pathogenicity of the bacterial mixture. Facultative organisms in mixed infections may provide a sufficiently reduced environment for the growth of obligate anaerobic organisms. Each component of the pathogenic mixture may contribute in different ways to produce the subsequent clinical picture. Experimental peritonitis in rats has led to observations that *E. coli* predominates initially in the peritoneal exudate. Bacteremia, the result of *E. coli* during the initial phase, is commonly present and frequently fatal. However, in rats that survive, indolent intra-abdominal abscesses develop in which B. fragilis predominantes. Elimination of the *E. coli* by early administration of gentamicin reduces early mortality, but does not prevent late intra-abdominal abscesses that result from the obligate anaerobes. In contrast, elimination of obligate anaerobes with clindamycin does not prevent early mortality caused by *E. coli* bacteremia, but does reduce late abscess formation in the survivors. These findings suggest that although *E. coli* is responsible for early mortality, anaerobes are responsible for the late abscess formation in the rat model.[11]

Thus, secondary peritonitis is typically polymicrobial, and the pathogens in the majority of patients are derived from gastrointestinal tract, even in patients with primary gynecologic trauma. Typically, the facultative microorganisms are *E. coli* and *Enterococci* and the obligate anaerobes are *B. fragilis, B. melaninogenicus, Peptococcus, Peptostreptococcus, Fusobacterium, Eubacterium lenteum,* and *Clostridium*. Primary management of intraperitoneal infection involves appropriate surgical drainage and debridement. Nevertheless, appropriate antimicrobial therapy can significantly reduce mortality among patients with intraperitoneal infections. Early use of appropriate antimicrobials is important if the inflammatory response and subsequent extent of damage is to be limited.[12]

Thus, the initial decision for antibiotic coverage must be empiric, and subsequent refinement will depend upon having obtained adequate aerobic and anaerobic specimens from the damaged tissue. These include cultures of the blood, as well as of peritoneal fluid. Observations have indicated that antibiotics need not be active against every pathogen isolated because a major role of the antibiotics is to reduce the replicative activity among microorganisms. The most important aspect of the host response involves the effective mobilization of polymorphonuclear leukocytes and macrophages as well as efforts to wall off infection through mobilization of the omentum in conjunction with fibrin and other exudative products. The management of intraperitoneal infections secondary to trauma involve the selection of an appropriate combination of antibiotics from among the overwhelming number of choices and combination of drugs available. I will highlight a few examples of commonly used antimicrobials that appear to be effective under most conditions. The goal is to select antimicrobials that are effective against gram-negative as well as gram-positive aerobic organisms and also effective against anaerobic organisms.

Aminoglycosides. Aminoglycosides have an excellent spectrum of activity against *Enterobacteriaceae* and *P. aeruginosa.* However, aminoglycosides hold no advantage over penicillins or cephalosporins against sensitive strains of organisms that may be causing the peritonitis. Because peak and trough concentrations may vary widely from individual to individual[13] and aminoglycosides in excess have been associated with ototoxicity, a decision to use aminoglycosides carries with it a decision to measure peak and trough values and maintain a very narrow therapeutic range between 4 to 8 μg/ml.

Penicillins. Penincillin G and ampicillin have excellent activity against all anaerobes, with the exception of *Bacteroides* species and *Fusobacterium* species. Ampicillin is usually active against the majority of strains of *E. coli* and the majority of *P. marabilis* strains. In addition, drugs like ticarcillin, mezlocillin, and piperacillin may be quite effective against anaerobes such as *B. fragilis.* Successful use of ticarcillin in combination with clindamycin or chloramphenicol has been reported for the management of intra-abdominal infections.[14] Finally, the combination of a B-lactamase inhibitor such as clavulanic acid, and penicillins such as ticarcillin has been reported to reduce the minimal inhibitory concentration of resistant strains of *B. fragilis* to low levels easily achieved by standard therapy.[15]

Cephalosporins. Cefoxitin is distinctly more active than cefalothin, cefamandole, or cefazolin against *B. fragilis.* In addition, it is also active against the majority of strains of *E. coli, P. marabilis,* and *K. pneumoniae.* Newer cephalosporins such as cefotaxime and ceftriaxone have demonstrated significantly better activity against the *Enterobacteriaceae* than the older cephalosporins. Ceftazidime has particularly good activity against *Pseudomonas* and is equal to other cephalosporins against the *Enterobacteriaceae.* However, it is only about one half as active by weight against gram-positive organisms as cefotaxime and has poor activity against *B. fragilis.* Thus, there appears to be no clearly advantageous role for any of the cephalosporins in the initial selection of antimicrobial coverage until specific organisms and their sensitivities are known. However, once known, cephalosporins may offer very specific advantages over drugs such as the aminoglycosides in that they are associated with far fewer toxicity problems, can be used in much broader therapeutic range, and generally have longer half-lives.[15]

Clindamycin. Clindamycin has been reported to inhibit over 95 percent of the anaerobes including *B. fragilis.* However, a few *Clostridium* strains, other than *C. perfringens, Peptococci* species, and rare strains of *Fusobacterium,* may be resistant. In addition, clindamycin is active against certain facultative gram-positive cocci, most notably *S. aureus and Streptococcus pyogenes,* but not *Streptococcus fecalis.* Clindamycin has virtually no activity against *Enterobacteriaceae.*

Metronidazole. Metronidazole is active against strict anaerobes and inhibits most *B. fragilis, Fusobacterium* species, *Clostridium* species, and has unique bactericidal action against *B. fragilis* and *C. perfringens.*[16] *In vitro* activity is poor against aerobes, microaerophils, and the anerobes, which may become somewhat aerotolerant on subculture. However, despite this poor *in vitro* activity, there is evidence that metronidazole has activity against *E. coli* in mixed aerobic–anaerobic infections.[17,18]

Chloramphenicol. Chloramphenicol has been demonstrated to have *in vitro* activity against over 99 percent of anaerobic pathogens involved in intra-abdominal infection. However, the *in vivo* experience with chloramphenicol has been not nearly as impressive as the *in vitro* susceptibility testing might predict. Two possible explanations involve, first, inactivation of chloramphenicol by products of resistant strains, and, second, a bacteriostatic impact rather than a bactericidal impact. Thus, despite the fact that chloramphenicol is easy to use and may even be reliably absorbed through oral administration, it is not a drug that should be considered as a first-line choice for the management of intraperitoneal infections.

Thus, the initial choice of antibiotics for the management of secondary peritonitis should include clindamycin at 25–40 mg/kg/day q 6–8 hr intravenously, in combination with gentamicin 3–7.5 mg/kg/day q 8 hr intravenously. Alternatively, metronidazole, 30 mg/kg/day q 6 hr, given in combination with an aminoglycoside is also appropriate initial therapy.[17,18] Once the organisms have been isolated and identified, appropriate substitutions of cephalosporins or penicillins for the aminoglycosides may be indicated by the results of *in vitro* susceptibility tests. Duration of therapy is usually prolonged to prevent relapse because host defenses cannot be relied on to eradicate completely the pathogens from sequestered areas of extensive necrosis and abscess formation.

Splenic Injury or Loss

The spleen is a major site of location of B-lymphocytes and is the major site for T-independent immune response mechanisms. Thus, intact splenic function is necessary for an individual to produce adequate antibodies to polysaccharide antigens.[19] In addition to its specific role in the humoral immune response reactions to polysaccharide antigens, the spleen also plays a major role by participating in the removal of opsonin-coated organisms and damaged cells from circulation. Thus, trauma to the spleen that necessitates splenic removal has been associated with subsequent risk of fulminant infections with encapsulated organisms such as *S. pneumoniae, H. influenzae* type b, and *Neisseria meningiditis.* In addition, there have been episodes of group A streptococcal infection among splenectomized patients. The greatest risk for fulminant infections appears to occur within three years post-splenectomy.

Not all post-splenectomy patients appear to be at risk for fulminant bacteremia. Those individuals who have underlying defects in serum opsonizing activity, or C_3 activation, or who make poor antibody to capsular polysaccharides appear to be in the major risk group for fulminant and overwhelming bacteremia. However, these humoral and complement defects are not normally measured and are reasonably prevalent in the population. Thus, it is appropriate to consider that all post-splenectomy patients should be considered at risk for fulminant bacteremia for a period of 3 to 5 years post-splenectomy.

Management of such patients has been controversial and there does not appear to be concensus in the literature. We now have polysaccharide vaccines against 24 capsular types of *Pneumococci, H. influenzae* type b, and *Meningococcal* strains other than type b. Response to these polysaccharide vaccines in the general population occurs best beyond 2 years of age and before the spleen is removed by at least 2 to 3 weeks. In contrast, the polysaccharide vaccines are probably of no value in children 18 months and younger and may be of unpredictable value in children who have been splenectomized. Nevertheless, it is the concensus that recently splenectomized children, if not already immunized, should be given immunization against the 24 capsular types of *Pneumococci,* as well as *H. influenzae* type b. Some recommend the use of daily penicillin V for up to 3 years post-splenectomy. This would appear to be appropriate, especially among children under the age of 2 years.

Pancreatic Injury

Prophylactic use of antibiotics early in the course of pancreatitis is ineffective in preventing subsequent development of pancreatic abscesses.[20] Therefore, the management of isolated pancreatic injury not associated with enteric spillage is primarily surgical, and involves repair and drainage.

Summary

Management of infections in children following traumatic injury must be approached with consideration for the age of the child and the dominant normal microflora of the injured area. Initial choice of antibiotic(s) should be broad and coupled with efforts to demonstrate the actual microorganisms involved. Once identified, specific antimicrobial choice can be made based on sensitivity data. Medical management, coupled with surgical drainage and debridement, leads to successful outcome where neither choice alone would otherwise be expected to succeed.

References

1. Goldstein EJC, Citron DM, Wield B et al: Bacteriology of human and animal bite wounds. J Clin Microbiol 8:667, 1978
2. Goldstein EJC, Citron DM, Finegold SM: Role of anaerobic bacteria in bite wound infections. Rev Infect Dis 6 (suppl 1):5177, 1984
3. Goldstein EJC, Citron DM, Gonzalez H et al: Bacteriology of rattlesnake venom and implications for therapy. J Infect Dis 140:818, 1979
4. Goldstein EJC, Citron DM, Finegold SM: Dog bite wounds and infection: A prospective clinical study. Ann Emerg Med 9:508, 1980
5. Elenbass RM, McNabney WK, Robinson WA: Prophylactic oxacillin in dog bite wounds. Ann Emerg Med 11:248, 1982
6. Bartlett JG, Gorbach SL: Anaerobic infections of the head and neck. Otolaryngol Clin North Am 9:655, 1976
7. Hand WL, Sanford JP: Posttraumatic bacterial meningitis. Ann Intern Med 72:869, 1970
8. Levine BA, Petroff PA, Slade CL et al: Prospective trials of dexamethasone and aerosolized gentamicin in treatment of inhalation injury in the burned patient. J Trauma 18:188, 1978
9. Pruitt BA Jr, Flemma RJ, DiVincenti FC et al: Pulmonary complications in burn patients: A comparative study of 697 patients. J Thorac Cardiovasc Surg 59:7, 1970
10. Hau T, Nelson RD, Fiegel VD et al: Mechanisms of the adjuvant action of hemoglobin in experimental peritonitis, Part 2. Influence of hemoglobin on human leukocyte chemotaxis in vitro. J Surg Res 22:174, 1977
11. Onderdonk AB, Bartlett JG, Louie T et al: Microbial synergy in experimental intra-abdominal abscess. Infect Immunity 13:22, 1976
12. Thadepalli H, Gorbach SL, Broido PW et al: Abdominal trauma, anaerobes and antibiotics. Surg Gynecol Obstet 137:270, 1973
13. Kaye D, Levison ME, Labovitz ED: The unpredictability of serum concentrations of gentamicin: Pharmacokinetics of gentamicin in patients with normal and abnormal renal function. J Infect Dis 130:150, 1974
14. Harding GKM, Buckwalk FJ, Ronald AR et al: Prospective, randomized comparative study of clindamycin, chloramphenicol, and ticarcillin, each in combination with gentamicin, in therapy for intra-abdominal and female genital tract sepsis. J Infect Dis 142:384, 1980
15. Neu HC: The new beta-lactamase-stable cephalosporins. Ann Intern Med 97:408, 1982
16. Ralph ED, Kirby WMM: Unique bactericidal action of metronidazole against *Bacterioides fragilis* and *Clostridium perfringens.* Antimicrob Agents Chemother 8:409, 1975
17. Aoki FY, Biron S, Doris PJ et al: Prospective, randomized comparison of metronidazole and clindamicin, each with gentamicin, for the treatment of serious intra-abdominal infection. Surgery 93(2):221, 1983
18. Stone HH: Metronidazole in the treatment of surgical infections. Surgery 93(2):230, 1983
19. Hosea SW, Brown EJ, Hamburger MI, Frank MM: Opsonic requirement for intravascular clearance after splenectomy. N Engl J Med 304:245, 1981
20. Ranson JH, Spencer FC: Prevention, diagnosis and treatment of pancreatic abscess. Surgery 82:99, 1977

CHAPTER 15

Community Responsibility for Pediatric Trauma Care

Burton H. Harris

S o much attention is paid to the untimely death of children from rare diseases that we sometimes forget that the leading health problem for children is trauma, which kills more children than all other diseases combined. Every year in the United States, 15,000 children die and another 100,000 are permanently disabled because of accidental illness or injury. Were an epidemic to cause a fraction of this death and disability, cries for action would be heard from all segments of society. But response has been curiously slow to the toll exacted by trauma—one of the most important public health issues in our country.

The trauma center movement has matured to the point at which legislative and regulatory bodies and insurance carriers are requiring the transfer of seriously injured patients to specialized facilities, where these exist. This coming of age poses special problems for those pediatricians and pediatric surgeons who have yet to commit themselves and their institutions to the care of such patients. Community involvement can be the catalyst for the creation of new systems of pediatric trauma care.

Trauma Care

Trauma care has six distinct phases: notification, pre-hospital care, transport, resuscitation, acute care, recovery, and rehabilitation. The design of trauma systems also involves preparation, education, and finance. The participation of members of the community is vital in each of these activities.

Notification

In urban settings, the amount of time that elapses between a medical event and receipt of the alarm by the emergency medical service is not a major factor in

Supported by a grant from the Kiwanis Foundation of New England mobilization of the trauma system. With the popularity of citizens band (CB) radios and, more recently, of cellular telephones, public safety agencies report an increased willingness of private citizens to report accidents and criminal activity. Cellular telephones have become so useful in some areas of the country that a national state police telephone number has recently been put into service.*

The situation in the rural United States is very different, and a road accident with victims who require medical assistance may go unreported for long periods of time. One solution to this problem is in use in rural Australia, where vehicles are now equipped with aviation-type transponders. Activated by the G-forces generated in crashes, the transponder sends a radio signal that is recognized by a satellite-based monitoring system, and a rescue unit is dispatched to the indicated location. Although this system could be used in any locale, public interest has not yet developed in the United States. Were the importance of "the golden hour" to achieve wide recognition, citizens might demand such an improved system of notification. Some localities might even begin to implement the "911" telephone-hotline system that has proven so valuable elsewhere.

Pre-hospital Care

The speed and effectiveness of field medical care is a major determining factor in survival after trauma. The work of Jacobs and associates clearly demonstrates the importance of airway control and maintenance of blood volume on eventual survival.[1] Appropriate pre-hospital care, measured by improvement in physiologic variables between the scene and the hospital, saves lives.

The political organization of American cities and towns virtually assures that every citizen has local police and fire protection. While the level of service varies, from volunteer squads and constables in some areas to highly organized and professional fire and police departments in others, these services are an accepted part of the tax base. Despite the Highway Safety Act of 1966, the concept of an emergency medical service as a third uniformed municipal force has yet to emerge in most localities. Although there are no private or proprietary policemen and firemen, pre-hospital medical care continues to be provided by private, for-profit ambulance companies in many major cities and rural counties.

This situation will not improve until change is forced by voters. Medical professionals can provide advice and professional direction, but the demand for quality pre-hospital care will be created by community expectations.

Transport

The care of seriously injured patients has become a highly skilled, technology-based medical and nursing specialty. Few of the thousands of community hospitals

---

*The national state police telephone number is 1-800-525-5555.

can do much more than stabilize an acutely injured patient; if a local hospital attempted to create a higher level of preparedness, it would in most instances be a misallocation of resources. More and more, when hospital staffs evaluate the commitment of equipment, personnel, and training that is required to care for trauma victims, they conclude that a referral plan is a more practical solution.

Triage—determining the destination of injured patients according to medical needs—is a prospective method for deciding the hospital to which a patient should be sent from an accident scene. When a choice exists, a patient should be taken to the hospital in which preparations and resources most nearly match care requirements. In recent years numerical scores have been shown to have predictive value for this task. The Trauma Score (TS), Revised Trauma Score (RTS), and Pediatric Trauma Score (PTS) all have been used for this purpose.[2,3] These severity indices make possible estimation of injury survival even before treatment has begun, and they are valuable triage tools.

Growth of the trauma center movement has been possible because of parallel developments in air and ground transport. As specialized medical care becomes increasingly regionalized, critical-care transport units are essential to move patients within the hospitals of the trauma care system.

The level of medical service that can be rendered in the field varies with the medical practice act of each jurisdiction. These laws define "medical control" and delineate the procedures that advanced emergency medical technicians (EMTs) and paramedics can perform. The experience of Cleveland and associates documents the surprisingly high level of diagnostic ability and therapeutic skill that pre-hospital personnel can attain.[4] Even though conspicuously successful pre-hospital systems have been operating for 20 years, some major states have yet to recognize any level of training beyond the basic EMT, while others prohibit paramedics from practicing life-saving measures known to be effectively used by their counterparts in other states. Improvements will come only from public pressure; involvement of the community in the form of advisory boards or representation on the governing bodies of transport systems will be necessary to effect change.

Aeromedical service became available in 1970 and has spread widely in the last two decades.[5,6] In the United States, the predominant model is the hospital-based helicopter in which a hospital critical-care environment has been replicated. The patient is attended by physicians, nurses, paramedics, and other medical specialists, and the aircraft becomes an extension of the hospital intensive care unit (ICU). Over 150 hospitals now operate more than 200 such aircraft, usually within the context of a regional system of referral medical care in which trauma is a significant component. As the financial climate for hospitals worsens, some of these services will become candidates for extinction. The community leaders who serve on hospital boards should be mindful of the contribution made by both air and ground transport, particularly in medically underserved areas, and act to preserve the advances of the last 20 years.

Resuscitation, Acute Care, and Recovery

The acute phases of trauma care are the responsibility of the first hospital to which the patient is taken, and the referral hospital to which some patients are transferred for definitive care. While community involvement does not extend into the resuscitation bay or operating room, it is community demand that makes such facilities available. Almost every hospital is controlled by a governing board representing the public. Public consciousness, political action, or market forces sooner or later influence directors of hospitals to provide trauma services.

The Resource Hospital

The hub of a pediatric trauma system is the tertiary care hospital, whose medical staff provides leadership and coordination and sets the standard of care. In regions in which a referral children's hospital exists, it should assume responsibility for pediatric trauma care. University hospitals with pediatric and surgical teaching services also can perform this service.

In the resource hospital, the pediatric trauma service should be an entity with a pediatric surgeon as the director, a geographic identity, separate budget, and representation on the medical board. Institutional commitment begins with a resolution of support from the hospital governing body, including an absolute guarantee of access to hospital services for pediatric trauma patients. The facility should publicize its willingness to accept all patients referred.

The major impact of providing care to pediatric trauma patients is seen in the emergency department, radiology department, operating room, ICU, and rehabilitation facilities. The laboratory must be capable of providing stat services on microspecimens, and the blood bank must be prepared to supply large volumes of blood and blood components on short notice. The presence of in-house physicians is a necessity.

The medical staff rules should require the admission of all children with injuries to two or more body systems to the pediatric trauma service for at least the first 24 hours of hospitalization. A pediatric surgeon is the single best physician to provide global care for these patients. Admission to a pediatric medical service because the patient is a child, or to a specialty surgical service because of a predominant injury, is inappropriate in an institution that is seeking to improve outcome. If pediatric surgeons are not present at the moment of admission they must become available promptly, because trauma is a surgical disease and the critical decisions, *especially decisions not to operate,* are surgical decisions.

Not every hospital should be a full-service trauma center. The attempt to achieve this would be unaffordable, and the medical specialty talent cannot be available around the clock. Modern trauma care depends on regionalization. Local hospitals agree to transfer patients in need of special expertise to a tertiary care center, and the referral hospital agrees to transfer the patient back when the need for special services has been met. A consensus must be reached in each hospital about what level of care can be provided, and a plan developed to assure availability of care in sister institutions. It sounds simple, but the decision by both sending and receiving hospitals to participate in such systems requires a high degree of commitment from the medical staff and the institutions' governing bodies. Such agreements are another example of community influence on medical decisions.

The concept of regionalization embraces community commitment to the system and support of the interdependent elements of the system. From agreement on system boundaries, provision of transport vehicles, and designation of the regional resource hospital, the cooperation of physicians, government officials, hospital administrators, and the public is necessary before any trauma system can provide reliable, efficient care.

Rehabilitation

The shortage in rehabilitation facilities is a true rate-limiting step in pediatric trauma systems. Not only is there a scarcity of physiatrists and rehabilitation centers, there is little specialization of personnel or facilities for the unique problems of children. However, many hospitals have rehabilitation programs, and post-trauma pediatric rehabilitation could be addressed by exportable programs sent home from the pediatric trauma centers for each patient.

Severity indices have recently been applied to the prediction of rehabilitation needs.[7] The National Pediatric Trauma Registry is the recipient of a grant for this purpose from the National Institute on Disability and Rehabilitation Research. An individualized arrangement for each patient is the goal of prospective severity scoring.

Educational rehabilitation and family counselling are as important as physical rehabilitation in preparing the severely injured child to resume a place in society. A recent followup study of pediatric trauma victims and their families documents the extraordinary and previously undescribed effects that serious injury has on patients, parents, and siblings.[8] These problems manifest in the areas of school adjustment, finances, and the integrity of the family unit. Social agencies, as the community resource to which families turn for help, often lack the expertise and special programs needed to deal with these problems. Only a demand for such services by a concerned public will encourage community agencies to plan for the care of pediatric trauma patients.

The involvement of volunteer hometown service organizations to meet the individual patient's needs on a case-by-case basis shows promise. The Kiwanis Clubs of New England, through their "Family Care Network," have rendered assistance by befriending programs during acute-phase hospitalization, and later by helping to prepare the child's home through renovation to remove physical barriers and by arranging for physical, occupational, educational, and emotional rehabilitation after the patient returns from the trauma center.[9] While not all families need this assistance, the program is a model of community involvement.

Trauma System Design

Activities that address design and finance of regional trauma systems and the educational and prevention aspects of child injury are beyond the scope of individual physicians and hospitals. By their nature, they are community problems and should be community decisions.

Do We Need a Trauma System?

The first hurdle in starting a pediatric trauma system is in achieving definition of the region to be served. In some places geography rules, but in others traditional patterns or unique circumstances may be more important. The identification of regional boundaries can be a sensitive issue and should be arrived at by consensus. While reaching agreement may be time-consuming and difficult, it is important because the borders of the region will dictate many operational details.

Once the limits and characteristics of the region have been defined, an epidemiologic study is required. The key data are an estimate of how many children are injured each year, which mechanisms of injury predominate, where the injuries occur, what facilities currently exist, and how many deaths might be preventable. Outcome goals should be established and compared with national norms. Because new relationships between hospitals will be necessary, the identification of institutions for the care of pediatric trauma patients is important, as is a working knowledge of existing transfer agreements and referral arrangements. While it can be laborious to gather these data, they are of great importance in designing a solution that truly fits the needs of the community. Conceptual errors at this stage are so fundamental that they will be difficult to correct later.

How Will It Work?

In addition to the quality of medical treatment, policy questions must be resolved. Regionalization means that patients will be transferred; who will decide when, where, and how? Numerical scoring systems and other schema based on mechanism of injury exist, as do less formal solutions. Transfer decisions can be made in the field, or the patient can be taken to the hospital nearest the accident and the decision made there, but a clear policy about transfer authority and criteria are essential. As long as perceived threats to reputation or economic well-being persist, the bypass of hospitals near an accident scene in favor of a designated hospital will be a constant and vexatious problem.

The mortar of an inter-hospital system is the transportation vehicles that move patients from one hospital to another. In most settings, both ground and air transport will be necessary. Within the system, the vehicles, hospitals, and EMS control agency should be connected by dependable communications. While different levels of care may be provided in various components of the transport service, an advanced life support (ALS) unit is essential for moving the most severely injured children to the regional referral hospital. In the last two decades, the principle has been assumption of responsibility for urgent critical care transport by the receiving facility, usually with hospital-based helicopters or mobile ICUs staffed by a doctor–nurse–paramedic crew.

While system design may appear to be a medical matter, these problems are rarely solved by doctors, and never by doctors working alone. Community support or resources may be appropriate to finance some aspects of the system. The real stimulus to formation of a trauma system is a social compact that acknowledges regional needs and brings the decision makers to the discussion table.

Education

Every trauma system has a public component and a professional component, and both need information. Public education begins with consciousness-raising. Although each year the United States loses more citizens to trauma than all the soldiers killed in the entire ten years of the Vietnam war, trauma remains a disease without a constituency. Emphasis on the problems of injured children, adults, and families should be given by government and the media, the two principal opinion-makers of contemporary society. The editors of newspapers and television news can make extraordinary contributions to trauma awareness and should become involved in the crusade. Community leaders and entertainment and sports celebrities have another level of influence that can help publicize the methods by which individual citizens can participate in the trauma system.

Very few health professionals currently in practice have received any formal training in pediatric trauma care. There are special techniques for treating child accident victims, and EMTs, emergency department physicians and nurses, physicians in the diagnostic and acute-care specialties, nurses, and others involved in the care of these patients need continuing education in pediatric trauma. Curricula have been devised and short courses developed for education at all levels.[10] Faculty can be drawn from the regional resource hospital and the courses presented at local hospitals or schools. These courses are essential in advancing the level and quality of care to be provided.

Finance

There have been profound changes in medical practice in the past few years. The next decade will see the shift from a needs-based to a cost-based system of care. New programs suffer in such an environment, especially programs with education, research, and prevention components which are not self-supporting. The solution lies in direct support from community involvement (Table 15-1).

Our experience with the establishment of the Kiwanis Pediatric Trauma Institute (KTI) has been an inspiring example of community in action.[11] A regional center for the study and treatment of pediatric trauma patients, KTI is supported by the 9000 members of the 253 Kiwanis clubs in Connecticut, Rhode Island, Massa-

---

Table 15-1. Sources of Funds for Trauma Centers

Hospitals
Patient fees
Community organizations
Corporations
Foundations
Private philanthropy
Government subsidy

---

chusetts, Vermont, New Hampshire, and Maine. Their support has made possible programs in education, research, patient care, accident awareness, and prevention.

The Kiwanis Pediatric Trauma Institute is a joint venture between the Kiwanis Foundation and the New England Medical Center. Its policy is set by an advisory board of physicians, hospital trustees, and Kiwanis representatives. Patients are accepted without regard to ability to pay; hospital and professional bills are paid by family medical insurance, automobile insurance, or public liability insurance. Patient care has been self-supporting, and free care and bad debt for the pediatric trauma patients has been very small, far below the percentage for the hospital at large. The Kiwanis donation supports education, research, and public affairs because these programs are not revenue-producing.

In other cities, alternate sources of outside support have been found for pediatric trauma centers. In Philadelphia and Pittsburgh, local foundations have embraced pediatric trauma care as a hometown issue appropriate for private sector concern. Substantial 3-year grants have been made to the Children's Hospital of Philadelphia and the Children's Hospital of Pittsburgh to seed trauma programs, and both have been quite successful. In Indiana, Michigan, and North Dakota, area Kiwanis clubs have pledged continuing support to local hospitals. In one memorable day in 1988, the Indiana District of Kiwanis raised $250,000 for the Trauma Life Center at Riley Children's Hospital in Indianapolis. In Charlotte, North Carolina, a prominent family with a long history of philanthropy endowed the Hemby Pediatric Trauma Institute at Charlotte Memorial Medical Center, and in Oklahoma City a public-spirited department store made a substantial donation to the Oklahoma Children's Memorial Hospital for a similar program. Two mature pediatric trauma services in Baltimore and Brooklyn are self-supporting with backup subsidy available from the host institution, one of which is a public hospital and the other a private institution.

As a group, each of these success stories share a common thread—a committed physician, an equally committed hospital, and an understanding community willing to start a joint venture to establish a new local resource. The usual donation or grant has been in the range of $150,000 to $250,000 per year for a 3-year period. The multiyear support aspect deserves emphasis because 12 to 18 months may be required to recruit key personnel and alter hospital systems before patients can be accepted. Even after initiation of service, interim financing is essential, because

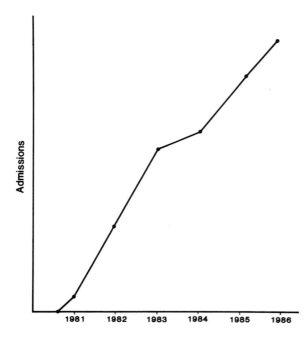

Figure 15-1. Trend curve for admissions to a pediatric trauma center for the first six years of operation. The slow initial period was followed by annual increases.

in most new programs more startup time can be expected before patient referral is established (Fig. 15-1). There also will be predictable times of relative inactivity (Fig. 15-2).

Extramural support usually depends on the provision of in-kind services by the hospital as a matching gift. Because tertiary-care hospitals already have the hardware necessary for the care of pediatric trauma patients, trauma centers are really a concept based on programs and people. In most instances, there is no need for new physical facilities. Donated money is misspent on ICUs, helicopters, beds, or durable equipment; it should be used to seed projects that attract new funds or to pay for otherwise unaffordable programs or services. Research grants are more easily available when joint institutional and community commitment can be demonstrated.

Summary

Modern trauma care begins at the moment of injury and ends with complete recovery. Total care includes rapid pre-hospital response, safe transport, community hospitals prepared to cope with pediatric trauma victims, the services of specialized referral centers for some patients, and a rehabilitation facility. When a plan integrates these clinical services with programs in education, research and public involvement, a trauma system exists.

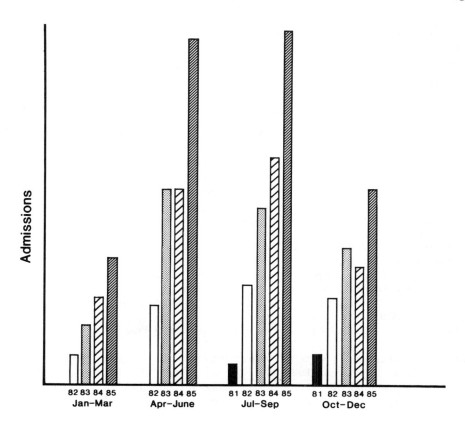

Figure 15-2. Seasonal distribution of admissions to a pediatric trauma center.

The goal for a regional pediatric trauma system is the provision of new and better medical care for pediatric accident victims. About 25 percent of those who are killed die unnecessarily, and countless others suffer permanent effects that may be equally avoidable. The development and impact of a pediatric trauma system depends on a coalition of concerned individuals and community organizations— doctors, nurses, parents, government officials, hospital trustees and administrators, business leaders, and service clubs—to define the methods by which we plan to eradicate this problem.

The importance of injury as the most important child health problem remains unrecognized. Unlike cancer, heart disease, muscular dystrophy, and other afflictions, trauma has no organized constituency and has faired poorly in attracting public attention or funds. Trauma remains an orphan disease that deserves to move higher on society's agenda.

We must resolve to commit ourselves and our institutions to respond to this public need. As a society and a profession we have yet to invest the time, talent, and resources to combat our biggest child health problem. How much longer can the health of our children be trusted to luck?

References

1. Jacobs LM, Sinclair A, Beiser A et al: Pre-hospital advanced life support—benefits in trauma. J Trauma 24:8–13, 1984
2. Champion HR, Sacco WJ, Carnazzo AJ et al: The trauma score. Crit Care Med 9:672–676, 1981
3. Tepas JJ, Mollitt DL, Talbert JL et al: Pediatric trauma score as a predictor of injury severity in the injured child. J Pediatr Surg 22:14–18, 1987
4. Cleveland HC, Miller JA: An air emergency service: The extension of the emergency department. Top Emerg Med 1:47–54, 1979
5. Cleveland HC, Bigelow DB, Dracon D et al: A civilian air emergency service: A report of its development, technical aspects and experience. J Trauma 16:452–463, 1976
6. Harris BH, Orr RL, Boles ET: Aeromedical transportation for infants and children. J Pediatr Surg 719–724, 1975
7. Gans BM, DiScala C: Are rehabilitation needs predictable? In Harris BH (ed): Progress In Pediatric Trauma, 2nd ed, pp 37–38. Boston, Nobb Hill, 1987
8. Harris BH, Schwaitzberg SD, Seman TM et al: The hidden morbidity of pediatric trauma. J Pediatr Surg 24:103–106, 1989
9. Lockwood DT, Harris BH: Family care in pediatric trauma. Emerg Care Quart 3:61–64, 1987
10. Harris BH, Murphy RE: Pediatric Trauma Management for Emergency Medical Technicians. Boston, Nobb Hill, 1987
11. Harris BH, Schwaitzberg SD: The Kiwanis Pediatric Trauma Institute. In Harris BH (ed): Progress In Pediatric Trauma, 2nd ed, pp 61–62. Boston, Nobb Hill, 1987

CHAPTER 16

Automobile Restraint Systems for Children

Kathleen Weber

A ll children riding in automotive vehicles should be protected from impact trauma through the use of appropriate restraining devices. Pediatricians and other health-care professionals often find it difficult to confidently guide parents on which of the many restraint types will best protect children of different ages, sizes, and physical conditions. Teaching parents to use these devices most effectively is an additional difficulty. This paper describes the theory behind the design of restraint systems, relates the principles to the various child-restraint systems available today, and presents some alternative restraint systems for children with special medical needs. For each type of restraint, we will also indicate the potential for injury from the restraints themselves (particularly when they are misused) and provide guidance for dealing with restraint use problems.

Restraint System Theory

In a motor vehicle accident, there are actually three collisions (Fig. 16-1). The primary impact is between the vehicle and another object. The second collision is between the occupant of the vehicle and its interior surfaces. The vehicle comes to a stop, but the passenger if unrestrained or loosely belted continues to travel forward. Third, there are collisions between the internal organs and the bony structures that enclose them. Restraint systems address the second collision directly, but also serve to mitigate the third type.

Crashworthy automobiles have not only a strong frame structure, but also a crushable sheetmetal structure that surrounds the frame. In a crash, the sheetmetal crumples, and cushions the impact for the part of the vehicle that is behind the crushing metal. This transfer of energy from the impact to the deformation of sheetmetal is called *energy absorption*. The front end of a car is a particularly effective energy absorber in a frontal collision because it folds up like an accordion, allowing the passenger compartment to come to a stop over a greater distance (and longer time) than the front bumper.

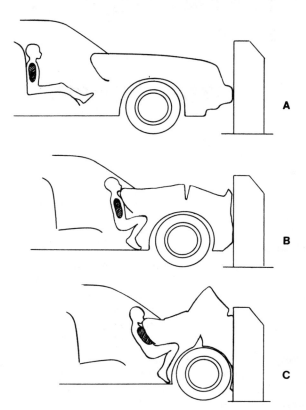

Figure 16-1. Three collisions: *A.* Vehicle to barrier; *B.* Occupant to vehicle interior; *C.* Thoracic organs to rib cage

Restraint systems are needed to extend the stopping distance of passengers and to minimize the contact between these passengers and the instrument panel or other interior surfaces. When securely tied to the frame of the vehicle through the use of a snug-fitting lap-and-shoulder belt, for instance, the occupant "rides down" the crash with the vehicle, rather than suddenly coming up against loosely adjusted belts or hitting the relatively unyielding interior at the vehicle's pre-crash speed. Controling the rate of the passenger's overall deceleration reduces not only the forces that act on the body surface, but also the differential motion between the skull and brain or the rib cage and the organs it contains.

However, reducing impact forces addresses only part of the problem. To optimize the body's impact tolerance, the remaining loads must be distributed as widely as possible over the body's strongest parts. For adults (who prefer to face the front of the car), this includes the shoulders; pelvis; and, secondarily, the thorax. For children, especially infants, alternate approaches are needed.

Proper placement and good fit are also important aspects of effective restraint systems. Serious restraint-induced injuries can occur when the belts are misplaced over body areas having no protective bony structure. Such misplacement of a lap-belt can occur during a crash if the belt is too loose or, with small children, is not held in place by a crotch strap or other device. This sliding of the pelvis under the belt is called "submarining." A lapbelt that is worn or rides up above the pelvis, can intrude into the soft abdomen and rupture or lacerate hollow and solid organs.[1] Moreover, in the absence of a shoulder restraint, the high lapbelt can act as a fulcrum around which the lumbar spine flexes, possibly causing separation of the lumbar vertebrae in a severe crash.[2,3]

The primary goal of any occupant protection system is to keep the central nervous system (CNS) from being injured. Broken bones will mend and soft tissue will heal with the help of surgical specialists, but damage to the brain and spinal cord is irreversible. In the design of restraint systems, it may therefore be necessary to put the extremities, ribs, or even abdominal viscera at some risk in order to ensure that the head and spine will be protected.

Child-Restraint Systems

There are several types of restraint systems designed especially for children. They vary with the size of the child, the direction the child faces when seated, and the placement of the vehicle seatbelt. All types, however, work on the principle of coupling the child as tightly as possible to the vehicle frame, and many provide additional energy absorption through padding or structural deformation upon impact.

There is an important difference between the restraint systems designed for infants and toddlers and those for older children and adults. The child-restraint carrier is anchored to the vehicle frame by the "adult" seatbelt provided in the vehicle, and the child is secured to the child restraint with a separate harness or other restraining surface (e.g., a shield). Therefore, it is critical that both the seatbelt and the harness be as tight as possible to provide the child with the best crash injury protection. If properly used and secured, child restraints reduce the risk of death and serious injury to their occupants by approximately 70 percent.[4] By comparison, estimates of fatality reduction to adults in lap/shoulder belts average about 50 percent.[5-7]

Infant Restraints

There are two types of restraint systems designed exclusively for infants. One places the infant facing the rear of the car. The other allows the infant to lie flat, perpendicular to the direction of vehicle travel.

Rear-Facing Restraints. In the United States, the most common restraint system for infants under 20 lb (9 kg) is a semi-reclined seat that faces the rear of the

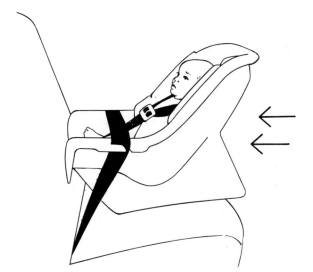

Figure 16-2. Rear-facing infant restraint showing direction of crash forces during frontal impact.

car. It is anchored in place with a seatbelt, and internal harness straps secure the infant's shoulders. In an impact, the crash forces are transferred from the back of the restraint to the infant's back, which is its strongest body surface, while the restraint also supports the infant's head (Fig. 16-2). Even in an off-center or side crash, the back of the rear-facing infant restraint swivels toward the direction of impact, still providing its occupant with effective protection. In rear-end and rollover crashes, which tend to be much less severe, the shoulder straps provide containment, and the restraint often rotates up against the vehicle seatback, completely enclosing the infant.

To work properly, the infant restraint *must* face rearward, and the harness straps must be over the shoulders and adjusted for a snug fit. If the infant's head or body needs lateral support, padding can be placed between the infant and the side of the restraint. Firm padding, such as a rolled towel, can also be placed between the infant and the harness strap or buckle between its legs to keep the infant's pelvis from sliding forward. Thick, soft padding should not, however, be placed under the infant or behind its back. Such padding will compress during an impact, leaving the harness straps loose on the infant's body.

Properly used, rear-facing restraints have proven to be extremely effective in actual crashes.[8,9] Unfortunately, parents and others who do not understand how an infant restraint is designed to work will often install it facing forward.[10] A laboratory test of this type of incorrect use with a popular infant restraint model indicates that there is a risk of serious neck injury from contact with the seatbelt, which is designed to hold the restraint in place, not the infant.[11] In this test, the shoulder straps

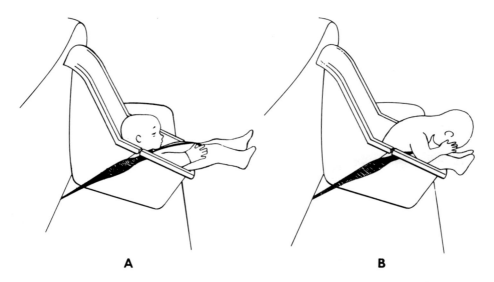

Figure 16-3. Infant and restraint during frontal impact, *incorrectly installed facing forward: A.* With shoulder straps in place; *B.* Without shoulder straps

were properly over the infant dummy's shoulders, so the dummy slid under the seatbelt until stopped at the neck (Fig. 16-3*A*). If these straps are not used, another common misuse, the dummy flexes at the waist around the lapbelt (Fig. 16-3*B*). When the belt is used to anchor the restraint in this incorrect orientation, it is too high and too far from the body to provide effective restraint. An infant in this situation would be likely to suffer spinal and internal abdominal injuries as its body is thrown into the seatbelt.

It is therefore critical that infant restraints be used facing the rear of the car. Two reasons that parents face infants the wrong way is that they are told over and over that the center of the rear seat is the safest seating position, and drivers like to be able to see their babies in the rear seat. This is especially true if the driver is the only adult in the car. Although the rear seat is a less hostile environment than the front seat and the center-rear position provides the most space between the child and the side of the car, it is "safest" only if all other factors are equal. Facing an infant forward in the back is worse than restraining the infant rearward in the front. In fact, rear-facing infant restraints perform very well in the front passenger seat, particularly when they rest against the instrument panel.[8] Some restraint models even have a slot in the back for the vehicle shoulder belt, so that it can help support the restraint in a crash (Fig. 16-4). If a driver wants to monitor an infant, the infant restraint should be placed rear-facing in the front seat, not forward-facing in the back.

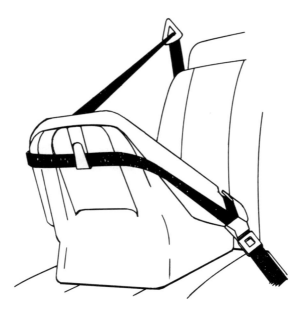

Figure 16-4. Rear-facing infant restraint secured with lap/shoulder belt.

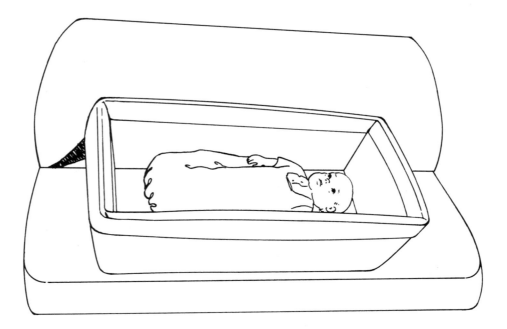

Figure 16-5. Infant car-bed restraint

Car-Bed Restraints. Another type of infant restraint is the car-bed or carry-cot (Fig. 16-5). This type is used more often in Europe and Australia, but is generating interest in the United States because of concerns about premature infants with positional apnea.[12] In a car-bed restraint, the infant lies flat, either prone or supine, and the bed is placed on the vehicle seat with its long axis perpendicular to the direction of travel. In a frontal crash, the forces are distributed along the entire side of the infant's body, while straps or a "baby bag," secured to the car-bed on each side with zippers, provide containment during rebound and rollover. In a side impact, however, the infant's head and neck are theoretically more vulnerable in a car-bed than in a rear-facing restraint, if the head is on the side nearest the impact. But crash experience with car-beds in other countries has not indicated a special problem with head or compressive neck injuries.[13,14]

Convertible (Infant/Toddler) Restraints

Convertible child restraints are designed to be used rear-facing for an infant and forward-facing for the toddler. The transition point is defined by the restraint manufacturer in terms of body weight, which is usually 18 lb, but may be as high as 20 lb. In reality, there is a considerable margin of safety built into convertible child restraints in the rear-facing position, and children would be better off facing rearward as long as they can comfortably do so, especially if the back of the restraint rests against the instrument panel. The designated "turn-around" weight for a restraint is not based on a careful, biomechanical evaluation of the tolerance of children to crash forces applied to the front of their bodies. Instead, its source is the 17.4 lb (8 kg) infant dummy used in the United States and Canadian standard crash tests of infant restraints and rear-facing convertible restraints weighs. Many manufacturers do voluntary tests with a 20-lb dummy. Thus, the weight selected in carrier restraint instructions may merely reflect the federal standard.

Case studies have identified 17 lb children whose injuries would have been avoided had they been facing rear rather than facing forward in convertible restraints at the time of the crash.[9,15] A case has also been described in which an 8-month-old child weighing "over 17 lb" escaped injury because he was restrained rear-facing when involved in a very severe frontal crash in a two-passenger sports car.[9]

While facing rearward, the shoulder straps should be left in the lower slots, regardless of the height of the child's shoulders, so that the straps can keep the child from ramping up the back of the restraint. Eventually, however, the parents will want to turn the restraint around to face forward. Although most parents want to make the transition much sooner, they should be encouraged to wait until the child is a year old and weighs 20 lb. The shoulder straps should then be raised to the higher slots, so that the strap forces press back against the shoulders and do not compress the shoulders and spine downward.

Restraint Design Choices. There are many different convertible child-restraint designs, and the public is understandably confused by the variety. Although all child restraints on the market today perform very well in crash tests and are very effective in protecting children in actual crashes,[4] differences among the internal restraining systems may affect a parent's choice.

The original strap arrangement in early child restraints was the 5-point harness, which was patterned after military and racing harnesses (Fig. 16-6A). There is a strap over each shoulder, one on each side of the pelvis, and one between the legs. All five come together at a common buckle. The function of the crotch strap is to hold the lap straps firmly down on top of the thighs, and thus it should be as short as possible. (Many child restraints in Europe and the United Kingdom do not have crotch straps, and their occupants are thus susceptible to submarining.[16,17] Because the crotch strap is merely a lap-strap positioning device, the primary lower torso restraint is still the combined lap straps. Although simple and effective, early 5-point harness systems were difficult to adjust and buckle around a squirming child, and complaints about twisting and "roping" of the straps continue today.

In the early 1980s, a creative designer replaced the lap portion of the harness with a padded shield (Fig. 16-6B). The shoulder straps were attached to the shield, which kept them straight, and could be more easily adjusted. The shield was still held in place by a crotch strap made of belt webbing. Other manufacturers quickly followed suit. Although these harness/shield combinations do not contact the body

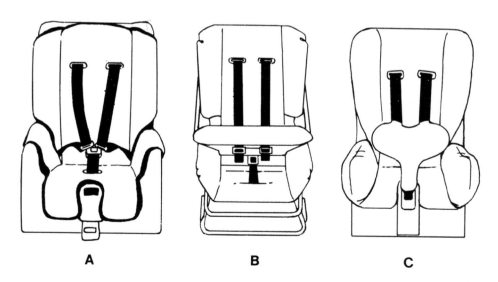

A　　　　　　　**B**　　　　　　　**C**

Figure 16-6. Convertible restraint configurations: *A.* 5-point harness, *B.* Harness/shield, *C.* T-shield

as low on the pelvis as the 5-point harness, they are much more convenient to use, and years of field experience have shown no performance problems.

About the same time, a Japanese manufacturer developed another variation on the 5-point harness that incorporated a retractor on the shoulder straps (Fig. 16-6C). These straps were attached to a flat chest shield with a relatively rigid stalk, which in turn attached to the child restraint between the child's legs. The overall shape of the shield and stalk has been compared to an elephant's head or bicycle seat and is often referred to as a T-shield. Eventually, similar designs began to appear on the U.S. market, some with automatic retractors and some with manual strap adjusters.

Although ease of adjustment and one-handed operation of the T-shield provide a further level of convenience for parents, there are some theoretical problems with this restraint configuration. Because the length and angle of the stalk is fixed, it is impossible to adjust the shield to fit close to a small child's body or low across the pelvis. The lower torso restraint of the lap belt is thus replaced by a narrow vertical stalk that concentrates impact forces at the center of the pelvis rather then spreading the forces across the pelvic breadth. Moreover, as discussed earlier, a loose-fitting restraining system does not couple the occupant tightly to the crushing vehicle, and higher forces on the body will result. Another concern is that the neck of a small child may be injured from contact with the top of the shield during a crash, especially in the forward-facing position. It is important to emphasize that these problems are, at the moment, only theoretical because we are not aware of any injuries related to use of this type of restraining system in actual crashes. In response to these criticisms, however, some T-shields have been designed or redesigned to make the stalk more flexible, to lower the height of the shield, and to provide two stalk attachment positions.

In recent years, easier means of adjusting 5-point harnesses have also been developed and are included on many of the newer models. Eventually, we hope to see 5-point harnesses incorporating automatic locking retractors, so that market demand will shift back to this inexpensive, lightweight, flexible, and effective restraining system.

Misuse and Injury Potential. There are a variety of ways to misuse a forward-facing child restraint. Incorrect routing of the vehicle belt has been well documented.[10,18] This can have anywhere from a minor to a disastrous effect on restraint performance, depending on the design and specific mis-routing.[11] Other commonly observed and dangerous practices include not using the harness straps at all, leaving the seatbelt or harness straps very loose, having the crotch strap very long, or placing the shoulder straps under the child's arms. Loose belts or straps will not couple the child tightly to the crushing vehicle, and higher crash forces on the body will result. A long crotch strap will place the lap straps up around the waist, where they may intrude into the soft abdomen during impact. Shoulder straps routed under the arms may crush or intrude under the child's flexible rib cage and cause serious injury to thoracic and abdominal organs. When the crotch strap is too long and the shoulder straps are under the arms, the child will flex around the straps at the waist, possibly causing fracture or dislocation of the lumbar spine and laceration of abdominal organs. These injuries would be similar to those produced by a lapbelt misplaced around a child's waist.

There has been some speculation in the past that a child's cervical spine could be pulled apart from the weight of the head in a crash when the shoulders are held back.[19] Although this may be true for an infant, who should be rear-facing anyway, it does not seem to be the case for children over 1 year of age. Several such cases have reached litigation, but when they are examined closely, there is always evidence of head contact occurring as the neck is in tension. This contact and sudden stopping of the head puts unnatural shear loads on the neck, which are the more likely cause of the fractures or dislocations. Unfortunately, those who document injuries in the medical literature are not usually in a position to also investigate the vehicle, the restraint, and the actual circumstances of the crash, and thus the true mechanisms of injury may be overlooked. However, several cases of severe frontal crashes in which fully restrained children have received no neck injury have been fully investigated and documented.[20]

Forward-facing convertible restraints are tested with a 3-year-old size child dummy that weighs 35 lb (16 kg) when fully instrumented with head and chest accelerometers. Nevertheless, most convertible child restraints claim to be for children up to 40 to 45 lb (18–20 kg). In practice, however, the limiting factor is usually the length of the harness straps, and, before the weight limit is reached, the restraining system cannot be buckled around the child.

Child Boosters

When a child can no longer fit into a convertible child restraint, the next step is a booster. Most boosters are not themselves restraint systems, but rather they depend entirely on the vehicle belts to hold the child and the booster in place. Thus they facilitate the transition between a child restraint and seatbelts.

There are actually two different types of boosters that have two different functions. The low-shield booster is designed to be used in a seating position with only a lapbelt (Fig. 16-7). It is the type most widely available today. The other type, which can best be described as a belt-positioning booster, is primarily designed to be used with a lap/shoulder belt (Fig. 16-8). It has small handles or hooks under which the lapbelt and the lower end of the shoulder belt are routed to position them better on a child's small body. The handles, functioning much like a crotch strap, hold the lap belt low and flat across the child's lap. The inboard handle also pulls the shoulder belt toward the child and makes its angle more vertical, so that it crosses the center of the child's chest. While low-shield boosters merely raise the child and transfer the lap belt load to a wide abdominal area, the belt-positioners adapt vehicle belt systems to a child's body size, so that he or she can take advantage of the built-in upper and lower torso restraint.

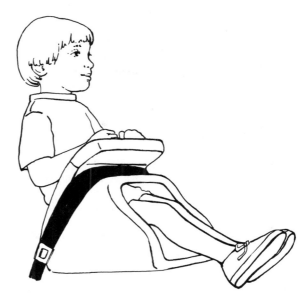

Figure 16-7. Low-shield booster

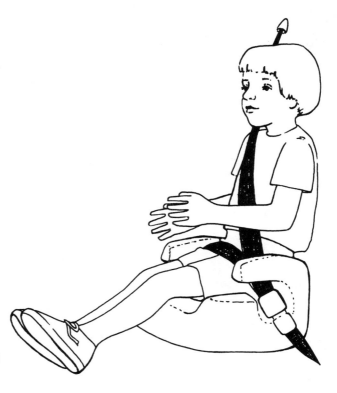

Figure 16-8. Belt-positioning booster

Booster Design Limitations. The original shield-booster (Fig. 16-9), which has a high shield rather than a low one, was developed in the mid-1960s.[21] The high shield acts much like an air-bag, restraining the head and upper torso in a frontal crash. This design was considered cumbersome and was often perceived as blocking the child's view. By lowering the height of the shield, however, all the impact forces are concentrated on the upper abdomen, rather than being spread over the entire front of the child's trunk. There are indications from laboratory tests of low-shield boosters with a specially instrumented dummy that these abdominal forces may be excessive, although we are not aware of shield-related abdominal or spinal injuries in the field.[22] Another advantage of the high shield is its ability to control head/neck motion and to protect the face during impact, which the low shield cannot do.

Although some low-shield boosters indicate in their instructions that a shoulder belt, if available, can be placed in front of the "taller child," this should be done with caution. The shield itself usually pushes the shoulder belt up and away from the child, making its angle worse with respect to the child's body. Moreover, the interaction between a shield restraint and a shoulder belt has not been thoroughly studied, and there are some indications that the two may be incompatible. The best approach at this time would be to place the shoulder belt behind a child, using a low-shield booster, as most instructions suggest.

The use of a belt-positioning booster with only a lapbelt is also not generally recommended. Without upper torso restraint, the more the child is raised off the vehicle seat the more the risk of head impact and consequent injury increases, owing primarily to the longer belt required to go around both child and booster.

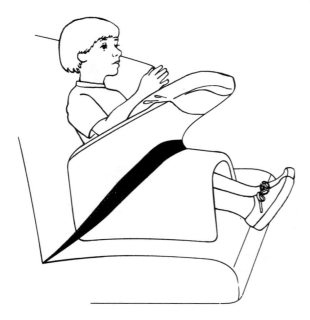

Figure 16-9. High-shield booster

As the belt is pulled tight during impact, the leading surface of the longer belt is higher and farther forward than the leading surface of a shorter belt that goes only around the child. The head of the child, whose body is rotating around this belt surface, will also travel farther forward than will that of an unrestrained child, allowing the head to hit interior surfaces that it otherwise would have missed.[11] With respect to head injury prevention, it is better for a child to sit directly on the vehicle seat when only a lapbelt is available than to sit on a belt-positioning booster. If, however, the lapbelt angle or seat contour is such that the belt will not stay low on the pelvis, and a more satisfactory seat and restraint combination is unavailable, it may be necessary to use the booster to prevent belt-induced spinal or abdominal injury.

Rear-Seat Lap/Shoulder Belts and Boosters. Although several models of the belt-positioning booster were manufactured in the early 1980s, parents were usually required to install a special set of child shoulder straps, because lap/shoulder belts were not generally available in rear seats where children sat. Now that rear-seat lap/shoulder belts are becoming standard equipment, these boosters are again becoming available to help provide effective, comfortable, and convenient restraint for children in the 3 to 7 year age range who ride in outboard front-seat and rear-seat positions. In addition, a new generation of booster seat has been developed that converts from one type to the other, depending on which type of belt system is available. These boosters have a low shield for use with a lap belt only, or the shield can be removed to leave belt-positioning hooks for use with a lap/shoulder belt. Of the two restraint configurations, the lap/shoulder belt with the belt-positioning booster is the preferred system because of its more effective upper-torso restraint and its better positioned lower-torso restraint. When used appropriately, however, both have performed well in actual crashes.

Boosters are only required to be tested with the 3-year-old (35 lb) dummy, but most manufacturers voluntarily test them with a larger 6-year-old dummy that can be weighted from 50 to 65 lb (23–30 kg). A child is too large for either type of booster, however, if his or her ears are higher than the top of the vehicle seat when the child is sitting on the booster base. When this occurs, the child will no longer be protected by the seatback from potential rear-impact neck injury. This height will vary from one vehicle to another and from front to rear seat.

Seatbelts for Children

There is no special age at which children "can wear seatbelts." Although vehicle seatbelts are designed with adult use in mind, they are not inherently unsuitable for children who can sit up unassisted. Seatbelts are part of a continuum of restraint systems with varying levels of effectiveness for children. In general, more restraint is better than less, and good fit is important for effective restraint performance. Child restraints typically have more restraining surface area (e.g., five straps or a broad shield) than does a lapbelt alone, and their restraining systems may be more easily positioned properly on a child's body. Good fit of a lapbelt is as low as possible on the pelvis or even flat across the thighs. A shoulder belt should cross the chest at mid-sternum and lie flat on the shoulder (Fig. 16-10).

Good fit for either a lapbelt or lap/shoulder belt is dependent on the size of the occupant, and suitable occupant size varies considerably from one specific belt-and-seat combination to another. Children should be restrained whenever possible by systems designed for their small bodies or by seatbelts adapted to their body size by a booster. However, if a child restraint or booster is unavailable, or if the child can no longer fit into one of these systems, then seatbelts must be used.

To achieve the best fit, the child should be sitting fully upright with his or her pelvis as vertical and as far back into the seat as possible. This will help place the lapbelt in front of the pelvic bone below the anterior-superior iliac spines, and which will minimize the possibility of the belt sliding up and intruding into the soft upper abdomen. The lapbelt must not be placed nor be allowed to ride up around the waist.

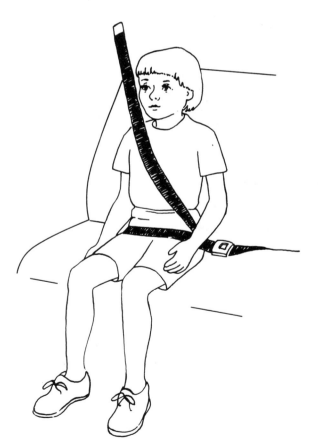

Figure 16-10. Properly positioned lap/shoulder belt

To place the shoulder belt away from the neck, the child should sit as close as possible to the side where the belt locks to the floor. Routing the shoulder belt behind the child is not recommended, unless the belt would otherwise have to lie flat across the throat or face. Shoulder belts that touch the side of the neck will not cause injury as long as they are snug on the shoulder.[23-25] Never place the shoulder belt under the arm of a child or adult because in a crash the resulting belt forces on the side of the rib cage are known to result in severe rib fracture and internal injuries.[26]

If a lap/shoulder belt can be made to fit the sitting child, it can be a very effective restraint system and is certainly preferred over the lapbelt alone. But the lapbelt should definitely be used if no other restraint system is available. For infants, however, there is really no effective alternative to the rear-facing or car-bed restraint.

Restraint Systems for Special Needs

Many children have special medical problems that preclude their being able to use standard infant or convertible child-restraint systems. These include premature infants who may be subject to oxygen desaturation in a semi-upright position, infants with Pierre Robin Syndrome (PRS), and children in various hip and body casts. In the past, health professionals and parents have been forced to see these children transported under unsafe conditions, either unrestrained or with potentially hazardous, makeshift systems. Recent research and development, however, have led to the availability of several restraint alternatives for these children. These alternatives and their availability will be covered briefly here because they are described in detail elsewhere.[27-30]

The car-bed was described above as an infant-restraint system in which the child lies prone or supine. Only one model, imported from Germany, is currently available commercially, and it has the disadvantage of being quite expensive. Although its standard-size restraining "baby bag" may be too large for a newborn, it can be replaced with a smaller bag available from another manufacturer. This car-bed is suitable for premature infants with positional apnea, infants with PRS, and children under 20 lb in flexed-hip or straight body casts. Other car-bed restraints are under development in the United States and should be available by 1991.

Another alternative for orthopaedic patients with flexed-hip casts is a convertible child restraint with cut-down sides and other modifications that allow the child to sit in the seat and be restrained by the harness straps (Fig. 16-11). These modifications do not affect the crash performance of the original child-restraint system. Although various models can be modified locally, there is one company that produces and sells child-restraint systems modified in this manner.

For children with straight body casts who are too long or heavy for the car-bed restraint, a body vest has been developed that allows them to be restrained lying flat across the vehicle rear seat (Fig. 16-12). The vest is made of seatbelt webbing; includes shoulder, chest, and pelvic straps; and is secured on one side

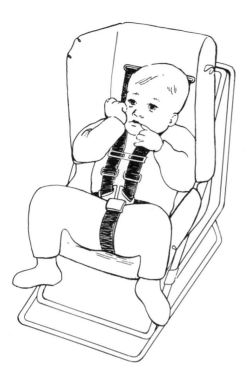

Figure 16-11. Convertible child restraint modified to accommodate child in flexed-hip cast.

with the vehicle's seatbelts. An additional strap at the knees secures the lower extremities. Although this restraint system is a significant improvement over no restraint at all, it does carry some risks. A side impact near the head could result in serious head/neck injury, and a frontal impact may produce intolerable lateral neck flexion. Padding at both the top and side of the head will mitigate these risks.

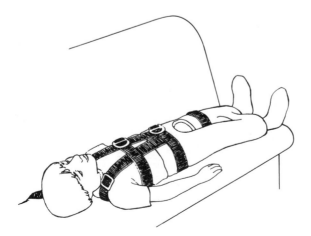

Figure 16-12. Body-vest restraint

Anatomic and Biomechanical Issues

Reference has been made above to a frequently cited paper by Burdi and associates on anatomic development in relation to child restraint design.[19] Although this work provides a thorough and valuable treatment of the body's structural and material changes from infancy to adulthood, many of its predictions about child injury causation under impact conditions have not been supported by actual field experience.[20,31] It has been found that, in general, children are less prone to injury than adults under the same impact conditions, and that the injuries they receive are less severe.

There is evidence that the more flexible thorax of the child reduces the risk of internal injury, because the ribs bend rather than break. Crash investigations also do not reveal that children are any more likely to submarine than adults, and serious neck injury is rare among all restrained occupants. Although the head is the most frequent injury site for all occupants, children do not suffer more severe injuries than adults, despite the fragility of their skulls. It is also not true that the unrestrained child will "lead with the head." A body free to move will travel in the direction of impact in the same orientation in which it was prior to impact. The mere fact that the head makes up a larger portion of the surface area of a child's body means that it is more exposed to contact. Finally, fears that small children will eject over the top of a lap belt, because of a high center of gravity, and that they will submarine under the belt, are contradictory. Evidence of the former has not been documented.

Regarding the apparent ability of children to withstand impact better than their adult counterparts, there is an easy explanation for restrained occupants that is often overlooked. The force on a body held by a seatbelt is directly proportional to the weight of that body. Specifically, $F = ma$, where m is the mass of the body and a is its negative acceleration, or its rate of reduction in speed as it comes to a stop. For example, a man weighing 180 lb (82 kg) riding down a crash at 15 G will experience a total force on his belts of 2700 lb (12 kN), while a 20-lb (9 kg) child in the same crash will experience only 300 lb (1.3 kN), spread over the restraint system. Even though the child's bony structure or soft tissue may be weaker than the adult's, the child's weight is so much less that the injury potential is less.

Unfortunately, there are only minimal data on the biomechanical response and tolerance of children to impact, and thus criteria for evaluating restraint systems are based on adult data. It would appear, however, that such criteria may be conservative. Thus currently available child restraints and seatbelts can be expected to provide at least as good, if not better, protection for children than seatbelts do for adults.

Conclusion

The consistent and proper use of restraint systems for infants and children in automobiles can prevent hundreds of deaths and thousands of injuries each year. Infants require the most special treatment, with restraint systems designed to apply crash forces to their backs or the full length of their bodies. Toddlers will also benefit from specially designed restraints that snugly conform to their small body shape, while providing elevation so that they can see the world around them. Seatbelts, too, can provide good restraint, even for young children, provided that attention is paid to good belt location and fit. With an understanding of both the theory behind the design of restraint systems and how this theory has been applied to child restraints, medical professionals who treat children and advise their parents will be better equipped to provide information about restraint systems, to encourage their proper use, and to deal with special restraint problems.

References

1. King AI: Abdomen. In Melvin JW, Weber K (eds): Review of Biomechanical Impact Response and Injury in the Automotive Environment, pp 125–146. DOT HS 807 042. Ann Arbor, University of Michigan Transportation Research Institute, 1985
2. Nyquist GW, King AI: Spine. In Melvin JW, Weber K (eds): Review of Biomechanical Impact Response and Injury in the Automotive Environment, pp 45–92. DOT HS 807 042. Ann Arbor, University of Michigan Transportation Research Institute, 1985
3. Taylor GA, Eggli KD: Lap-belt injuries of the lumbar spine in children: A pitfall of CT diagnosis. American Journal of Roentgenology 150:1355, 1988
4. Kahane CJ: An Evaluation of Child Passenger Safety; the Effectiveness and Benefits of Safety Seats. DOT HS 806 890. Washington, DC, National Highway Traffic Safety Administration, Feb 1986
5. Evans L: The effectiveness of safety belts in preventing fatalities. Accid Anal Prev 18:229, 1986
6. Huelke DF, Sherman HW, Murphy M et al: Effectiveness of current and future restraint systems in fatal and serious injury automobile crashes. SAE 790323. Warrendale, Pennsylvania, Society of Automotive Engineers, 1979
7. Partyka SC: Belt effectiveness in fatal accidents. In Papers on Adult Seat Belts— Effectiveness and Use. DOT HS 807 285. Washington, DC, National Highway Traffic Safety Administration, June 1988
8. Melvin JW, Weber K, Lux P: Performance of child restraints in serious crashes. Am Assoc Automotive Med Proc 24:117, 1980
9. National Transportation Safety Board: Child Passenger Protection against Death, Disability, and Disfigurement in Motor Vehicle Accidents. NTSB SS-8301. Washington DC, Sep 1983
10. Cynecki MJ, Goryl ME: The Incidence and Factors Associated with Child Safety Seat Misuse. DOT HS 806 676. Southfield, Michigan, Goodell-Grivas, Dec 1984.
11. Weber K, Melvin JW: Injury potential with misused child restraining systems. SAE 831604. Stapp Car Crash Conf Proc 27:53, 1983
12. Willet LD, Leuschen MP, Nelson LS, Nelson RM: Risk of hypoventilation in premature infants in car seats. J Pediatr 109:245, 1986
13. Bowler M, Torpey S: An Evaluation of the Victorian Baby Safety Bassinet Loan Scheme. Hawthorn, Victoria Road Traffic Authority, July 1988
14. Czernakowski W: Comments on car-bed experience in Germany. Ulm, Romer-Britax, 19 Oct 1988
15. Diekema DS, Allen DB: Odontoid fracture in a child occupying a child restraint seat. Pediatrics 82:117, 1988

16. Conry BG, Hall CM: Cervical spine fracture and rear car seat restraints. Arch Dis Child 62:1267, 1987
17. Lowne R, Gloyns P, Roy P: Fatal Injuries to Restrained Children Aged 0–4 Years in Great Britain 1972–86. Crowthorne, Transport and Road Research Laboratory, 1987
18. Shelness A, Jewett J: Observed misuse of child restraints. SAE 831665. In Child Injury and Restraint Conference Proceedings, pp 207–215. Warrendale, Pennsylvania, Society of Automotive Engineers, 1983
19. Burdi AR, Huelke DF, Synder RG, Lowrey GII: Infants and children in the adult world of automobile safety design: Pediatric and anatomical considerations for design of child restraints. J Biomech 2:267, 1969
20. Dejeammes M, Tarriere C, Thomas C, Kallieris D: Exploration of biomechanical data towards a better evaluation of tolerance for children involved in automotive accidents. SAE 840530. In Advances in Belt Restraint Systems, pp 427–440. Warrendale, Pennsylvania, Society of Automotive Engineers, 1984
21. Heap SA, Grenier EP: The design and development of a more effective child restraint concept. SAE 680002. New York, Society of Automotive Engineers, 1968.
22. Melvin JW, Weber K: Abdominal intrusion sensor for evaluating child restraint systems. SAE 860370. In Passenger Comfort, Convenience and Safety, pp 249–256. Warrendale, Pennsylvania, Society of Automotive Engineers, 1986
23. Appleton I: Young Children and Adult Seat Belts: Is It a Good Idea to Put Children in Adults Belts? Wellington, New Zealand Ministry of Transport, Road Transport Division, Aug 1983
24. Corben CW, Herbert DC: Children Wearing Approved Restraints and Adult's Belts in Crashes. New South Wales, Traffic Accident Research Unit, Jan 1981
25. National Transportation Safety Board: Children and lap/shoulder belt use. In Performance of Lap/Shoulder Belts in 167 Motor Vehicle Crashes, vol 1, pp 63–71. Washington, DC, Mar 1988
26. States JD, Huelke DF, Dance M, Green RN: Fatal injuries caused by underarm use of shoulder belts. J Trauma 27:740, 1987
27. Bull MJ, Weber K, DeRosa GP, Stroup KB: Transporting children in body casts. J Pediatr Orthop (in press), 1989
28. Bull MJ, Weber K, Stroup KB: Safety seat use for children with hip dislocation. Pediatrics 77:873, 1986
29. Bull MJ, Weber K, Stroup KB: Automotive restraint systems for premature infants. J Pediatr 112:385, 1988
30. Indiana University, Automotive Safety for Children Program: Safety Home. (videotape.) Indianapolis, Riley Hospital for Children, 1988
31. Newman JA: The Restraint of School-Age Children in Automobiles: A Literature Review. Ottawa, Biokinetics, Oct 1979

Preventing Childhood Injury in the United States: The National SAFE KIDS Campaign

Martin Eichelberger

I njury is the leading cause of death among children in the United States. Annually, 8,000 children are killed by preventable injuries, another 50,000 are permanently disabled, and 10,400,000 children sustain injuries that require emergency room treatment. One in three children will sustain an injury that needs medical attention; one in five will require hospitalization. Despite the severity of this situation, social ignorance and misunderstanding are hampering efforts to make injury prevention a priority in American life. The traditional view persists that injuries are the unavoidable outcome of unfortunate circumstance. This cultural prejudice has restrained scientific investigation and the development of effective preventions and treatments and has blocked their widespread implementation. Former U.S. Surgeon General Dr. C. Everett Koop has described the contradiction eloquently, "If a disease were killing our children in the proportions that accidents are, people would be outraged and demand that this killer be stopped."

But public opinion and the allocation of public resources have not caught up with the reality that most injuries can be prevented. A 1987 survey by Peter Hart & Associates showed that parents were far more concerned about the threat to their children from abduction and crime (47%) or drugs (43%) than from injury (32%). The current federal health research budget allocates 14 times more money to cancer and heart disease than to injury—although injury causes the loss of more years of potential life before age 65 than cancer and heart disease combined.

National SAFE KIDS Campaign

The National SAFE KIDS Campaign is designed to reduce childhood injury through alteration of the ways Americans live and care for children. This task involves transformation of ingrained cultural values and habits of personal behavior, as well as modification of products and environments and the institutionalization of injury-prevention programs.

Mission

The SAFE KIDS Campaign mission is to reduce the number of fatal and nonfatal injuries to children.

The Campaign has targeted the five highest injury risk areas for children: motor vehicle, bike, and pedestrian accidents (43.3%); burns (15.3%); drowning (14.9%); poisoning and choking (3.5%); and falls (2%). Six objectives form the focus of the five-year Campaign.

1. Sponsoring grassroots activities to develop national commitment to injury prevention
2. Collaborating with voluntary and governmental agencies to increase spending on injury prevention
3. Stimulating activities to implement changes in environments, products, laws, and behavior that will prevent injury to children
4. Participating in the strengthening of existing injury-prevention programs and organizations and initiating programs where none exist
5. Supporting the Surgeon General's Health Objectives on injury prevention for 1990
6. Focusing attention on children of low-income families who have been statistically demonstrated to be at higher risk

Targets

The Campaign seeks to reach three groups: children, parents and other caregivers, and persons in a position to change public policy.

There are two goals related to children, parents, and other caregivers. Obviously, the first goal is to change individual behavior so as to decrease the likelihood and severity of childhood injury.

The second, equally important goal is to mobilize the widest possible participation of children, parents, and caregivers in advocacy work for injury prevention—that is, to enlist their active support in local coalitions. For instance, at recent Senate hearings Christopher Clark from Connecticut made a moving plea for bike helmet use. Clarke was permanently disabled at age 14 by a head injury sustained in a bike accident. A helmet would have prevented this injury. There are many individuals who can offer compelling testimony on the necessity and validity of injury-prevention efforts. Further, public pressure is an important ingredient in the range of activities required to secure effective changes in public policy.

The third target group consists of persons in a position to change public policy. *Product manufacturers and trade associations* can set safety standards for design and production. *Legislators* can enact laws mandating product safety standards or establishing requirements of public behavior (such as wearing seat belts), and also designate funds for injury prevention research and programs. *Public health administrators and other public officials* can set policies that raise the priority of injury prevention. Because of the difficulty of influencing individual behavior on a mass scale, it is vital that organizing efforts reach this key group.

Organization and Financial Support

The SAFE KIDS Campaign is a creative partnership that draws upon the diverse energy, expertise, and resources of hundreds of organizations nationwide that are concerned with childhood injury prevention. A long-term effort, initiated in 1987 by Children's Hospital National Medical Center (Washington, DC) the Campaign receives major funding from the Johnson & Johnson Company and additional support from the National Safety Council. The organizational foundation of the Campaign is the National Coalition to Prevent Childhood Injury (NCPCI), which consists of over 60 national organizations focusing on children or those who care for them.

A Technical Advisory Board, composed of injury prevention, medical, and health and safety experts, reviews Campaign plans, provides programmatic guidance and direction, and plays an important role in Campaign evaluation. A Public Policy Committee draws on the expertise of NCPCI member organization and elected officials at all levels of government. The Committee formulates initiatives to secure manufacturer product safety standards; funding support for injury programs or research; improvements in the environments of children; and legislation that mandates behavioral, product, and environmental changes. The National SAFE KIDS Office in Washington, DC, coordinates media and public policy work, develops educational materials, and facilitates the development of local, state, and national coalitions.

Key to Success

The key to the success of the SAFE KIDS Campaign has been establishing local and state coalitions. By its second year, the Campaign had built over 60 local coalitions in 35 states. These are the heart of the Campaign, setting the tone for its efforts and ensuring genuine contact with parents and children in each community. Much more than just a local "presence," the local coalitions serve several important functions.

Draw together diverse segments of a community. These can include injury-prevention specialists, medical professionals, educators, communicators, legislators, businesses, business leaders, and civic organizations. This concentration of effort inevitably propels an increase in local injury prevention activity. For instance, in numerous cities, local organizations hired new staff specifically to work on SAFE KIDS. Also, the emergence of local coalitions often attracts local financial sponsors. These have included Hallmark Cards, AMOCO, Grand Union Stores, local drugstore chains, and local Chambers of Commerce.

Localize the focus for their community. Often the safety emphasis in one community will differ from that in another, and the Campaign facilitates the most targeted approach possible. For example, in St. Louis, the local campaign is built around the theme of "wheels"—skateboards, bicycles, and traffic safety. In Alabama, the effort is aimed at raising the age requirement for the state's child restraint law.

Generate publicity at national and local levels. USA Today ran a full-page article on the SAFE KIDS Campaign because of the Campaign's local coalitions and nation-wide activities in cities. The local television coverage generated by National SAFE KIDS Week is invariably the result of local coalition activities. It was the existence of the local coalitions that moved the National Association of Broadcasters and radio and television stations in more than 25 media markets to join the SAFE KIDS Campaign.

Act as a distribution point for educational materials and information. The local coalitions consistently request materials to support their activities. As demonstrated during the 1988 National SAFE KIDS Week, coalitions educate and inform through safety fairs, bike rodeos, and other activities, reaching people through schools, clubs, retail outlets, and other community distribution points. In its first year, mainly through coalition members nationwide, the Campaign distributed more than 1.5 million free injury-prevention booklets, *"How To Protect Your Child From Injury.*

Serve as primary vehicle for achieving community-based improvements in child-hood injury-prevention. Some coalitions have lobbied hospitals to ensure consistent use of the injury data collection system known as "E-Codes." Some have met with school officials on introducing injury-prevention education into the school curriculum, and others have worked to ensure that childcare workers are taught CPR. It is the local coalitions that have the clout and ability, socially and politically, to achieve changes in product safety, legislation, environments, social awareness, and education.

It is the creation and facilitation of the local coalitions that distinguish the National SAFE KIDS Campaign in its efforts to change public attitudes and action. Without this grassroots base, the national Campaign could be little more than a massive public relations effort. While National SAFE KIDS builds momentum among key organizations, policy makers, and the media, it also guides local coalitions in implementing their injury-prevention campaigns based on local conditions. The local coalitions make actual progress in injury prevention, thus providing the national effort with basic content and credibility.

The first National SAFE KIDS Week in May, 1988, was officially opened by President Ronald Reagan, who publically signed the SAFE KIDS Week Proclamation in the White House Rose Garden. Dr. C. Everett Koop, Surgeon General of the United States, was the Campaign's Honorary Chairman. Both honors were in recognition of the Campaign's nationwide presence in coalitions on the local level.

The existence of the local coalitions also facilitated acceptance of SAFE KIDS as a "Bulletin Campaign" by the Ad Council. The CBS and ABC television networks aired SAFE KIDS public service announcements over a period of two months. Articles were placed with several syndicates and wire services—including AP, UPI, and the *Mini Page*—and in several national magazines, including the Sunday supplement *Parade, USA Today, U.S. News and World Report, Parenting, Children's Magazine, American Baby,* and *Sesame Street.*

In just over 10 weeks, the Campaign generated more than 72,000 calls to its toll free number. In addition, then Secretary of Defense Frank Carlucci sent a memo to all branches of the armed services requesting their participation in SAFE KIDS Week and stressing the importance of increased injury-prevention activities. It is clear that his directive was implemented—the Army and Navy each ordered 180,000 parent's booklets.

Celebrity involvement has also helped to gain support for the campaign.

Methods

To accomplish its objectives, the SAFE KIDS Campaign implements a multi-faceted campaign. It is the integration of these approaches—at the local and national levels—that gives the Campaign its dynamic quality. Each prong of the SAFE KIDS strategy affects the others. By pursuing all fronts simultaneously and in an interconnected fashion, SAFE KIDS maximizes its abilities.

Public policy initiatives endeavors to influence the laws, regulations, and institutionalized policies that influence childhood safety in the community. A good example from the Campaign's work in Year I is the voluntary agreement of the Gas Appliance Manufacturers Association (GAMA) to preset all newly built water heaters at 125° F, a temperature low enough to prevent hot water scalding in children. Another example is the Senate hearings in February, 1989, which were initiated by Senator Christopher Dodd (D-CT) and designed to identify areas in which federal legislation could enhance injury prevention in the United States.

Media work includes efforts to increase through radio, television, and print exposure the general public's awareness of injury prevention: the problem, risks, resources, and ongoing prevention activities.

The Campaign aims to counteract the prevailing media coverage of injuries, which focuses on the horror of injury and fosters a sense of tragedy and hopelessness. SAFE KIDS emphasizes to the media that most injuries are not simply accidents—they have specific causes and can be prevented.

Community action is carried out by the local and state coalitions. Each coalition is made up of community groups such as local departments of health, safety councils, children's hospitals, firefighters, women's clubs, and church groups. These public-service-minded organizations unite to implement the local efforts to reduce injury.

Education is conducted to provide people with information on childhood injuries and how to prevent them.

The Bike Helmet and Bike Safety Awareness Campaign

In 1989, the SAFE KIDS Campaign conducted a nationwide bike-helmet and bike-safety awareness campaign that concentrated on implementing all the experience gained in Year I.

Local coalitions continued to plan and implement the injury-prevention programs most appropriate to their local situations, but they were also given the opportunity to introduce the national-level campaign on bike helmets and safety. In some cases, the national focus amplified local effort; in others, it provided a context for the establishment and development of a local coalition.

Bike Injury Focus

Bike injuries were chosen as the focus for the 1989 National SAFE KIDS Campaign for two reasons. First, it is a problem of significant magnitude. Every year over 380,000 children are injured in bike-related incidents and require emergency room care. In bicycle collisions with motor vehicles, 400 children under age 15 are killed and another 37,000 are injured. The number of bicycle injury deaths has increased by 27 percent in the last 10 years. Second, research by private and governmental organizations has pinpointed the ways in which all types of bicycle injuries happen. This understanding defines the logical areas for intervention programs and in many cases outlines what type of intervention would be most effective. Knowing how bicycle injuries occur also provides prevention activists with convincing arguments to use in outreach efforts.

Helmets

The central issue in bicycle injury prevention is helmet usage. More than 75 percent of pediatric bike-related deaths involve head injuries. One in 7 children under age 15 will suffer a head injury in a bike crash. One third of child cyclists who are in an accident require emergency room treatment, and two thirds of those hospitalized have head injuries. A recent Seattle study indicated that helmet use could prevent the majority of deaths and disabilities that are caused by head injuries.

No studies have documented current helmet use among children; it is thought to be minimal, about 1 or 2 percent. However, it has been demonstrated that helmet use can be increased significantly through concerted community-based campaigns. In Seattle, the Harborview Injury Prevention and Research Center and the Washington State Society of Pediatrics spearheaded a campaign that increased helmet use to 16 percent in two years. In Victoria, Australia, a four-year campaign increased helmet use among children commuting to elementary school to 69.7 percent. The elements of these successful campaigns have been adopted for use in the national SAFE KIDS program.

Bike Helmet Campaign

The popularity of cycling has doubled since 1970. The number of bicycles in use is now 111 million, and an array of organizations to serve bicycling interests have been created. These cyclist organizations are especially concerned about head injuries and have formed the HeadSmart coalition, which also launched a bike helmet campaign in 1989. The HeadSmart coalition—which includes the National Head Injury Foundation, the American Academy of Pediatrics, the Bicycle Federation of America, and National SAFE KIDS—are collaborating in a powerful organizational effort to reach a broad audience through a unified safety message.

This type of campaign makes it easy for local communities to get involved, while ensuring that local efforts will be augmented by national attention and resources. Experience has shown that successful bike helmet campaigns can be conducted by organizations and coalitions of various sizes. Never has it been so easy to have an effective impact. The emergence of a coordinated effort between the cyclist and the safety communities raised hopes that a significant gain can be made in bike helmet use in 1989 throughout the United States.

Bike Safety Awareness

While the possibility of severe head injuries would seem reason enough for wearing a helmet, most parents are unaware of the frequency with which they occur and have never considered making their children wear a helmet when bicycling. After all, the great majority of parents never used a helmet and never suffered head trauma.

This lack of understanding makes it necessary to convince parents that while bicycling is a relatively risky activity, children can ride in reasonable safety if they follow safe cycling rules and wear helmets. Thus, the central message, "wear a helmet every time you ride a bike," is framed by an all-rounded bike-safety theme that identifies the major risks for cyclists and informs parents and children of the skills and behavior that can be used to counter each risk. The high-risk situations are riding out into the street, suddenly swerving into traffic, "wrong-direction" riding, and careless riding at intersections.

Targets

The targets of the bike-helmet campaign were 5 to 10-year-old children and their parents (or other caregivers). Education began with 5-year-olds because this is the age when children begin to ride bicycles. From 5 years up to about age 8, most children recognize that bicycle riding is difficult and dangerous, if only because while learning to ride they frequently wobble, fall, and have trouble stopping. They are susceptible to a safety message. Around age 7, children begin to ride in streets and encounter increased danger. Their confidence in their own skills is rising, but they face new situations with which they are not familiar—street signs and signals, rules of the road, and riding in traffic. By age 10, peer pressure makes it difficult to convince a youngster who has not yet done so to wear a bike helmet. At this point helmets are not considered "cool."

It is important that parents and other caregivers set the standard for bike safety and helmet use. Parents should not let their children ride without wearing helmets and following safety rules, regardless of the conduct of other parents and children.

When bicycle riding themselves, parents always should wear a helmet. Preschools should supply helmets for toddlers who play on tricycles, and schools should require helmets for children who commute by bike. As these behavioral norms are established, children will grow up with new expectations and will be able to resist any lingering peer pressure against helmet use.

Reaching Parents and Kids

The primary way to reach children and parents about bike safety and helmets is through small group presentation and discussion. This method was the focus of the educational component of the 1989 SAFE KIDS Campaign. To facilitate local organizing efforts, the national staff prepared presentation outlines, a helmet Q&A list, visuals suggested for use, handouts for parents and kids, and a poster. Parents and children were contacted through hospitals, PTAs, church groups, women's clubs, youth groups, service organizations, and schools.

Local coalitions launched their campaigns with "bike-skills rodeos" and strong media campaigns. A bike-skill rodeo is designed to teach skills and reveal weaknesses, by showing how injuries happen. In a "fun" atmosphere, the rodeo focuses community attention on bike safety and provides opportunities to promote helmet use (helmets are required for participation, and "loaner" helmets are provided).

The focus on bike safety and helmets provided specific opportunities to expand the local SAFE KIDS coalitions among bicycle retailers and bike clubs. The Campaign's specific focus on bicycle safety acted to draw certain schools, PTAs, youth groups, businesses, and service organizations into the effort.

Helmet Availability, Cost, and Quality

An element critical to the widespread use of bike helmets is their availability and cost; helmet quality is a related issue.

Currently, many outlets that sell children's bicycles do not sell helmets, and others do not promote helmet sales. Still others do not sell helmets that meet the performance standards of the two private organizations that evaluate helmet safety, the American National Standards Institute (ANSI) and the Snell Memorial Foundation.

Moreover, because the instance of helmet use is so low, sales are low and production runs among manufacturers are small. Thus, prices are relatively high and can approach half the cost of the bicycle itself. Helmet manufacturers are small businesses that do not have a manufacturers association nor the resources to advertise or promote helmet use. For the most part, they are not prepared to meet any sudden increase in demand for their product.

For these reasons, it was important that the SAFE KIDS Campaign work with helmet manufacturers to secure their cooperation in the bike helmet campaign. The Campaign alerted the manufacturers that the campaign was being planned and would increase demand for their product. At the same time, price reductions were negotiated to encourage helmet purchases and accelerate the pace of initial sales. It was also necessary to negotiate with manufacturers so that they would market their helmets through selected children's bike retailers as the campaign moved into high gear over the spring and summer. This was to counteract the problem of most good quality helmets being sold exclusively in bike specialty shops.

In addition to helmet availability, the SAFE KIDS national staff wanted to ensure the quality of helmets. Thus, one public policy component of the Campaign was to pursue the establishment of a national bike-helmet safety standard with the Consumer Products Safety Commission and the U.S. Department of Transportation.

Lessons of SAFE KIDS Injury Prevention Organizing

The bike helmet campaign—particularly SAFE KIDS' cooperation with the Head-Smart coalition and the support and encouragement provided to local initiatives—will carry forward in Year II the principles established and lessons learned in the highly successful Year I of SAFE KIDS. These principles have broad application.

Respect existing programs, people, and organizations already involved in injury-prevention activities. Bring such people and groups together to develop cooperative initiatives. They have gained a wealth of experience through previous activities, and can offer valuable knowledge of organizations and the political terrain. SAFE KIDS can serve to stabilize and establish organizational alliances among injury-prevention activists that have been years in the making. One of the main contributions SAFE KIDS can make to injury prevention is to give the reason, excitement, and support for organizations to build the coalitions they've always wanted to form.

Look for new energies and resources that can be tapped for injury control. Efforts in the past have been limited too often to health and professional medical organizations. But the issue of childhood injury prevention will elicit interest and support from diverse organizations. Local SAFE KIDS coalitions are being sponsored by drugstores, Rotary Clubs, Chambers of Commerce, and a variety of small businesses. Energetic support has been given by the Boy Scouts, 4-H, Women's Auxiliaries of the VFW, the General Federation of Women's Clubs, Kiwanis Clubs, police departments, and the military, to name just a few.

Work in concert with coalition members' agendas. Don't be afraid that individual coalition members will use the coalition for their own purposes. Analyze how individual interests coincide with the coalition's agenda. Given the voluntary nature of the coalition, organizations will only contribute to the degree that the coalition activity serves their own purposes, but this need not be a negative factor. Boy Scouts want to keep down injuries in Scout activities; Red Cross chapters and Safety Councils want people to call on them for safety services; hospitals want people to think of them not only as care providers but also as advocates for children's health and safety; businesses want potential customers to see them as positive community partners; and politicians want votes. If the united activity of a SAFE KIDS coalition is drawing media attention to the issues of injury prevention, and funds and energy are being focused on a bike helmet campaign or housing safety regulations, the goals of the coalition are being addressed.

Allow for different kinds of participation while clearly designating a lead agency and lead group to guide the coalition's work. Inevitably, different organizations have different expertise and amounts of time and resources to devote to the campaign. Recognize a multi-faceted strategy genuinely requires the expertise of a public relations person. What distinguishes SAFE KIDS coalitions from places where there are only SAFE KIDS activists has been the commitment made by one organization to be the lead agency, and the most successful SAFE KIDS coalitions have organized three to six core organizations into a steering committee. Successful coalitions are simultaneously loose and tight—loose in their openness to different kinds of participation by members—tight in the organization of a leading group to direct energies to clear objectives.

Expect ebbs and flows in the activities of a coalition. Every coalition goes through many stages, from the initial period of excitement and high energy to the scary, sometimes disheartening periods of questioning if goals can be met, if organizations can work together, and dealing with organizational structures to the times of refocusing on more realistic objectives and implementation of specific plans. A coalition cannot function in high gear all the time; members have many other demands on their time. Plans need to take into account the ebbs and flows. It's better to do a small number of activities well and accomplish specific goals than to experience the frustration of not meeting unrealistic expectations.

Facilitate the possible. The art of effective coalition activity is a clear assessment of what is really possible. The whole point is to maximize and build upon that assessment. The success of efforts to sustain coalition activity will come down to how well expectations and action agendas fit with the actual interests and capacities of coalition members. Experience has proven that realistic expectations mobilize tremendous collective energy and open unprecedented avenues to childhood injury prevention at the community level.

Our Children's Time Has Come

Children have moved onto center stage on the United States' agenda for the 1990s. Failures in the past have made it clear that it is far better to invest in our children now than to wait and pay the social cost later. Childhood injury prevention is an important aspect of creating the best possible future for our children and, thus, for our society. It's hard to say no to the SAFE KIDS Campaign. In fact, everyone wants to be involved. Through the Campaign, we are making a big difference in American life and culture. The SAFE KIDS campaign is leading the way into a new era in which childhood injury, like smallpox and polio, will no longer be a major threat to the quality of children's lives.

CHAPTER 18

Pediatric Trauma in South Africa

Sidney Cywes, Shelley M. Kibel, and David H. Bass

I njury is the major cause of death and disability in South Africa between ages 5 and 34 years and accounts for 36 percent of all years of potential life lost.[1] As is the case in many developing countries, data on pediatric trauma in South Africa, especially morbidity, are not readily available. It is necessary to compile a general picture from isolated studies, a tactic that does not add up to a representative picture of the country as a whole. Statistics on injury-related mortality represent the only fairly reliable nationwide injury data available in South Africa, although they do not give a complete picture of the problem.

This chapter outlines the population structure, sociocultural background, mortality, and morbidity of injuries (both accidental and intentional) in South African children under age 15 years and discusses the major categories of injury in more detail. Injuries and patterns of injury that are peculiar to South Africa are highlighted, and the steps that could be taken to prevent them are considered.

Sociocultural Background

South African society is diverse, divided, and complex and has features resembling both developed and developing countries. In 1985, the population was estimated at 27.7 million,[1] excluding the four independent national states of Transkei, Bophuthatswana, Venda, and Ciskei (TBVC). The population is classified into four racial groups: Blacks, Coloureds (people of mixed racial descent), Asians, and Whites, with each group living in specified areas. Of the total population, 76 percent are Black, 14 percent White, 8 percent Coloured, and 2 percent Asian.[1] Thirty seven percent of the total population are children under 15 years of age (10, 272, 900), which is 40.7 percent of the Black group (7, 759, 200), 35.5 percent of the Coloured (1, 016, 900), 32.3 percent of the Asian (278, 300) and 24.6 percent of the White group (1, 218, 500).[1]

Demographic, sociological, environmental, and behavioural factors that influence society contribute to the complexity and scope of the injury problem.[2] The effects of the sociocultural and political changes on the family have been well documented.[3,4] Industrialization, rapid urbanization, a migratory labour system, and Westernization have resulted in the loss of traditional lifestyles. Increased unemployment, uncontrolled population growth, lack of housing, violence, and civil disturbance have affected poor families and their children, who are more vulnerable and exposed to the hazards of injuries. Many differences in the patterns of childhood injury among population groups are related to socioeconomic factors and not to ethnicity, although cultural factors do play a role. There is substantial evidence from other countries that socioeconomic factors influence the incidence of injuries.[5-7]

Injury-Related Mortality

The available mortality statistics are based on registered deaths,* which are known to be low estimates, especially in the Black population.[8,9] The Black population is also underestimated in the population census. For these reasons, it is impossible to calculate accurate mortality rates for the total population. To assess the relative importance of the different causes of injury deaths, the proportional mortality has been calculated for the whole population.

In most developed and many developing countries, injury is the leading cause of death in the 1 to 24 year age group.[10] In South Africa, the majority of all childhood deaths are caused by infectious diseases (primarily measles), gastroenteritis, perinatal causes, respiratory disease, and malnutrition and these still play a major role in the under-5-years age group (Table 18-1). After 5 years, injury becomes the major cause of death, accounting for 43 percent of all deaths in the 5 to 14 year age

Table 18-1. Rank Order and the Proportion of Major Causes of Death Under 15 Years of Age, RSA - 1981–1985*

Rank Order	Under 1 Year	%	1–4 Years	%	5–14 Years	%
1	Infectious	33	Infectious	42	Injury	43
2	Perinatal	31	Respiratory	17	Infectious	14
3	Ill-defined	14	Ill-defined	13	Ill-defined	13
4	Respiratory	13	Injury	11	Respiratory	9
5	Congenital	3	Endocrine	11	Nervous system	7
Average annual deaths	24, 112		8, 512		3, 611	

*Unpublished data. Institute of Biostatistics (Medical Research Council) and Child Safety Centre, University of Cape Town

---

*Registered deaths are classified by the Central Statistical Service, Pretoria, according to a system based closely on the "International Statistical Classification and Causes of Death (ICD), 1975." Prior to 1978, the 8th Revision was used and after this the 9th Revision (see Appendix).

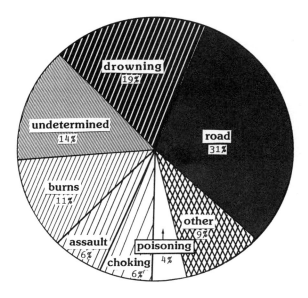

Figure 18-1. Pie diagram showing the major causes of injury-related mortality in children under 15 years

group. In White children the pattern is similar to that found in Western developed countries. The injury rates for White, Coloured, and Asian children from 5 to 14 years old have not changed much since 1968, although there has been significant year-to-year variation. As in other countries, more boys die of injury-related causes than girls.

The major causes of injury-related mortality in children under age 15 years are shown in Figure 18-1 and the average number of injury-related deaths in each population group are presented in Table 18-2. The ICD codes included in each

Table 18-2. *Average Number of Injury Deaths Under 15 Years Per Year by Cause and Population Group, RSA: 1981–1985*

	Blacks	*Whites*	*Coloured*	*Asian*	*Total*
Road	458	151	218	41	868
Drowning	326	92	121	7	546
Burns	234	12	51	7	304
Assault	114	18	46	4	182
Choking and					
suffocation	83	3	41	4	166
Poisoning	85	7	18	2	112
Other	153	33	58	3	247
Undertermined	276	41	59	20	396
TOTAL	1,729	392	612	88	2,821
TOTAL POPULATION UNDER 15 YRS[1]	7,759,200	1,218,500	1,016,900	278,300	10,272,900

cause group are shown in Table 18-3. All external causes are included (E code). Overall, road-traffic-related injuries are the major cause of injury mortality, followed by drowning, injuries that may have been accidental or deliberately inflicted, and burns. Each population group has a unique pattern of incidence (see Table 18-2).

The causes of injury probably vary among areas of the country and especially between urban to rural areas. For example, in one study of non-natural deaths, based on medicolegal autopsies in Cape Town, Knobel and associates found that 54 percent of these deaths were from road traffic injuries, 13 percent from burns,

Table 18.3. ICD E Codes Used in Analysing Injury Mortality Statistics (Includes all External Causes: E800–E999)

E Code Definition	8th Revision	9th Revision
Road traffic (motor vehicle) injuries	810–827	810–829
Drowning	910	910
Burns:		
Fire	890–899	890–899
Scalds	924–926	924–926
Assault:		
homicide	960–969	960–969
legal execution	970–978	970–978
war-related	990–999	990–999
Choking + suffocation	911–913	911–913
Poisoning, accidental	850–869	850–869
Injuries, undetermined if accidentally		
or purposefully inflicted	980–989	980–989, 889*
Other:		
Transport other than	800–807	800–807
motor vehicles	830–838	830–838
	840–845	840–845
	927	846–848
Mines	937	849
Falls, accidental	880–887	880–888
Nature	900–909	900–909
Machinery		919
Struck by	916–918	916–918
Sharp instrument	920	920
Firearms, accidental	922	922
Sport	939	839
Iatrogenic	930–936	870–879
	947–949	930–949
Suicide	950–959	950–959
	979*	979*
Miscellaneous	914, 915	839, 914, 915
	919, 921	921, 923
	923, 929	927–929
	940–946	

*Additional codes used by Central Statistical Services, Pretoria

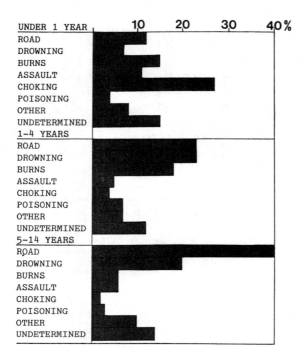

Figure 18-2. Distribution of injuries by age (< 15 years)

11 percent from drowning, 5 percent from assault and 3 percent from poisoning.[11] As in other countries, the distribution of causes of injury varies considerably with age (Fig. 18-2).

Morbidity

For every childhood death from injuries, there are many more children who suffer injury, some of whom will be permanently disabled. An injured South African child may be treated in any one of a wide range of institutions—from rural clinics to accident units in teaching hospitals—depending on the severity of the injury and the geographic area where it occurred. No national trauma registry or injury surveillance systems exist in South Africa, and apart from statistics regarding road accidents, hardly any national data describing childhood injuries have been assimilated. However, statistics of nonfatal childhood injuries are provided, based principally on data from the Red Cross War Memorial Children's Hospital (RXH). These are not representative of the country as a whole. Red Cross Hospital is situated on The Cape Peninsula, which has a population of 1.6 million[1] of which 750,000 (47%) are children under the age of 15 years. Since April 1984, all injured children presenting to RXH have been managed in a pediatric trauma unit.

Table 18-4. Causes and Nature of Injury in Children Under 13 Years Presenting to RXH Trauma Unit January 1986 to December 1987: Nature of Injury

Cause of Injury	Soft Tissue	Burns	Head Injury	Musculoskeletal	Foreign Bodies	Trunk Injuries	Total
MVA pedestrian	773	3	1,064	413		175	2,428
MVA passenger	109		171	57		25	362
MVA other	175	1	143	82		17	418
Bumps and blows	1,824		1,208	524	28	294	3,878
Sharp instruments	1,199			2	27	15	1,243
Assault	246		234	48	4	79	611
Burns		3610				7	3,617
Falls	2,537		4,033	3,038	5	568	10,181
Animal bites	578				1	4	583
Others	264		156	170	896	157	1,643
Total	7,705	3614	7,009	4,334	961	1,341	24,964

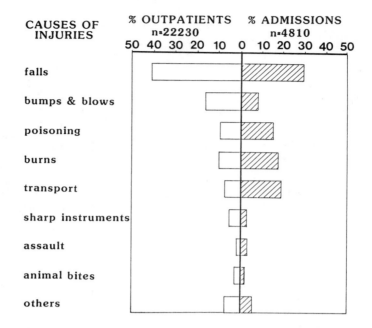

Figure 18-3. Causes of injuries treated as out-patients and as in-patients in the Trauma Unit at Red Cross Children's Hospital

Causes of Injury

From January 1986 to December 1987, 24,099 children presented to the RXH pediatric trauma unit with a total of 24,964 injuries. In addition, 2,871 children were managed for acute poisoning and near-drowning. The causes and types of injury are shown in Table 18-4 and the causes by out-patient and in-patient care are shown in Figure 18-3. Over the 2-year period, trauma accounted for 3 percent of all hospital out-patient visits and 11 percent of all admissions.

Falls were the most common cause of injury, being responsible for 70 percent of musculoskeletal injuries, 56 percent of head injuries, and 33 percent of soft-tissue injuries. The majority of fall injuries were minor, having occurred on level ground, from beds, or from the arms of a caregiver. Although falls were the most common cause of injury in patients requiring admission, this finding differs from that of the Paediatric Trauma Centre at The Johns Hopkins Hospital, where falls accounted for half as many admissions as motor vehicle accidents (MVAs).[12]

Bumps and blows ranked second as a cause of injury, but in contrast with American[13] and Canadian[14] studies, sports-related injuries were uncommon. This may be attributable to the age-limit of 13 years.

Burns were responsible for even more injuries than MVAs, and accounted for almost as many trauma admissions. This contrasts sharply with both the United Kingdom,[15] where burns and scalds are responsible for barely 5 percent of all domestic injuries and North America,[13] where burns constitute less than 3 percent of all injuries. Burns were also the third most common indication for trauma admissions at RXH and will be dealt with separately in this chapter.

Transport-related injuries, although constituting only 12.8 percent of all accidental trauma, accounted for most of the multiple injuries requiring intensive care (99 in 2 years), and in-hospital deaths from to trauma (42 in 2 years). MVAs have also been shown to be the most common cause of severe head injuries in children who require hospital admission in Cape Town.[16]

Assault included a total of 611 case, with 112 cases of alleged rape and 309 patients in whom chronic abuse or neglect was suspected. Children with physical or sexual abuse seen in the trauma unit constituted 60 percent of all abuse cases at RXH.

Road Traffic Injuries

The leading cause of childhood injury mortality in South Africa, as in other countries,[17] is road-traffic injury. From 1981 to 1985, 64.7 percent of such deaths involved passengers in motor vehicles, 34.9 percent were pedestrians and only 0.4 percent were cyclists.[18] However, the proportion of pedestrian deaths varies considerably by age and population group. In the United States, injuries to pedestrians account for 39 percent of MVA-related deaths under 15 years of age.[19]

Table 18-5 shows the age, sex, and cause of specific annual mortality rates for road traffic injuries in South Africa for 3 population groups and compares them to other developed and developing countries.[10] These comparison figures are averages of 5 developed countries outside Europe and 17 developing countries, mostly in Latin America. Rates for the Black population group have not been estimated for reasons previously stated. The road-traffic mortality rates in White, Coloured, and Asian children are exceedingly high when compared to both developed and developing countries. This applies especially to the Coloured population group, where South African rates are up to 5 times greater than the average in other developed or developing countries. The age 5 to 9-year group had the highest rates, and the rate for boys exceeds that of girls. The MVA-related death rate for American children under 15 years was 6.6/100,000 in 1984.[19]

Road-traffic injury is the only injury cause for which national morbidity data are available. Compared with Australian[20] and North American[14] studies, bicycle MVAs were uncommon, constituting 8 percent of all injuries and 3.1 percent of deaths from road accidents.[21] Passenger and pedestrian MVAs were responsible for 90 percent of all South African transport injuries in children under 15 years for 1986.

There is no doubt that misuse of alcohol holds a significant responsibility in

Table 18-5. Age, Sex, and Cause-Specific Annual Mortality Rates* for Three South African Population Groups and Comparison Countries 1981–1985 (Per 100,000 Population)

| | South Africa | | | | | | Developed Countries[10] | | Developing Countries[10] | |
| | Whites | | Coloureds | | Asians | | | | | |
	Boys	Girls	Boys	Girls	Boys	Girls	Boys	Girls	Boys	Girls
< 1 year										
Road	17.22	11.56	12.19	11.21	14.74	4.49				
Drowning	8.35	4.40	14.62	4.98	4.21	2.24				
Burns	2.09	0	14.63	11.21	2.11	2.24				
1–4 years										
Road	12.55	10.04	24.43	18.89	15.17	10.66	8.1	6.6	5.5	4.1
Drowning	25.84	13.25	20.16	12.1	1.57	1.6	9	4.8	7.1	4.8
Burns	1.61	1.55	10.59	7.68	7.32	5.33	4.6	3.4	4	3.5
5–14 years										
Road	15.05	10	26.78	17.58	17.39	13.2	8.5	4.7	7.4	4
Drowning	4.23	1.72	15.31	5.49	3.68	1.86	3.7	0.8	4.6	2.1
Burns	1.13	0.25	2.85	2.24	1.23	1.03	1.2	1.1	0.8	1.3

*Unpublished data. Institute of Biostatistics, Medical Research Council and Child Safety Centre, University of Cape Town, 1989 (Central Statistical Services enumerated population data were used in calculating these rates.)

the high rate of road-traffic deaths. The legal blood alcohol limit is 0.08 g/mL in South Africa, compared to 0.05 g/mL in most Australian states.[22] Secondly, despite compulsory use of seatbelts having been introduced in 1977, seatbelt legislation and enforcement have only recently come into effect. Since 1964, all new cars have had to be fitted with front seatbelts, and rear seatbelts have been required since 1987. Although the specification as to type and installation of infant and child seatbelts and chairs have been approved and adopted there is no legal enforcement for their use. A third factor responsible for the high pedestrian injury rate, especially in urban areas, is the paucity of playgrounds in Coloured and Black neighbourhoods, where streets are used as playgrounds.[23]

Motor-vehicle-related injuries are the major cause of head and thoracoabdominal injury admissions. These serious injuries are discussed in more detail later in this chapter.

Head Injuries

Since the RXH trauma unit opened in 1984, head injuries from blunt trauma have been the most common indication for admission. The majority of these are minor, resulting from falls, especially in children under age one year. Overnight admission to hospital is indicated for logistic reasons as often as for medical reasons because many families live considerable distances from the hospital and have poor access to transport. Sixty percent of severe head injuries in patients aged 1 to 14 years resulted from MVAs, one half of which were pedestrian MVAs.[16] Consequently, many of these patients suffered multiple injuries. As shown in a previous study, however, in-hospital mortality was directly related to the presence and severity of head injury alone.[12] Our experience with head injuries is difficult to compare with those published by other centers because definitions of "severe head injury" and admission criteria vary from study to study. It is notable, however, that in one study from the United Kingdom, MVAs were responsible for only one third of the head injuries that required admission in all children under age 15 years.[24]

Our management of head-injured children does not differ significantly from that of other units. The majority of these patients are cared for in the trauma unit itself, but children who require assisted ventilation are nursed in a pediatric surgical intensive care unit (ICU). The vast majority of patients are treated conservatively.

Little data, except from retrospective studies, exist on the long-term sequelae of childhood head injuries.[25] If unrecognized, even the most subtle neurological impairment after minor head injury may have disastrous long-term implications, especially for a child whose chances of a normal education and productive life are already handicapped by socioeconomic disadvantages. In 1984, a Cape Town Head Injury Study Group began to study prospectively the outcome of all head-injured children admitted to RXH. Only in such a way can the true morbidity of these distressing injuries be assessed.

Thoracoabdominal Injuries

Because of the high prevalence of blunt trauma, predominantly from MVAs, closed chest and abdominal injuries are frequently seen at RXH. Since April 1984, 106 children with *blunt chest injuries* have been treated, almost exclusively the result of MVAs.[26] The most common injuries sustained were lung contusions, rib fractures, and hemothoraces. All patients had at least one other injury. Conservative management, consisting of continuous intravenous morphine infusion and drainage of intrapleural collection has been successful in all patients with blunt chest trauma, and there have been no septic complications of intercostal drainage. Penetrating chest injuries have been uncommon, amounting to no more than 3 cases per year.

The spleen is the organ most commonly injured as a result of blunt abdominal trauma.[27] However, over an 11-year period (1978–1988), 228 *liver injuries* were encountered, all resulting from blunt trauma. The value of nonoperative management of pediatric liver and spleen injuries has been described by ourselves and others.[28–30] Only 8 of 228 children with liver injuries underwent laparotomy, 5 of these being indicated for extrahepatic intraperitoneal injuries. One child required emergency laparotomy on day 6 for a ruptured subcapsular hematoma. There were no other complications related to conservative management.

Over the same 11-year period, 96 *splenic injuries* were encountered, of which 84 responded well to nonoperative management. Nine of these patients underwent laparotomy for suspected hollow viscus injury, which was confirmed in only 2 cases. Laparotomy was performed in 3 patients who had signs of ongoing hemorrhage, but only 2 splenectomies in total were performed.

A nonoperative management policy for 203 *renal injuries* (1984–1987) has also been adopted with a resulting nephrectomy rate of 1.5 percent. Laparotomy was required in 9 patients for assorted injuries.

Radionuclide scanning (RNS) has been relied upon principally for the confirmation of liver and spleen injuries, and conventional intravenous pyelography is used for diagnosis of renal injuries. Whole-body computed tomography (CT) has been available since June 1987, but has been found to be less sensitive than RNS, particularly in the detection of minor lacerations and contusions. We prospectively studied 45 patients with blunt abdominal trauma and clinical signs of intra-abdominal bleeding.[31] Each patient underwent abdominal CT and RNS. The RNS studies revealed 29 liver and 13 splenic injuries in 35 children. Only 5 of the liver injuries and none of the splenic injuries were detected by CT. Although this confirms the findings of other reports,[32] it is possible that our diagnostic yield from CT may improve with greater experience.

Compared with solid organ injuries, *hollow viscus injuries* are relatively uncommon. Over the last 11 years, we have performed laparotomy on 29 patients who sustained hollow viscus injuries as a result of blunt trauma (20) and penetrating trauma (9). A further 13 patients underwent laparotomy for penetrating abdominal trauma over the same period and no viscus injury was found. Repeated clinical examination of these patients has been found to be the mainstay of diagnosis, and plain abdominal roentgenograms were singularly unhelpful in all but 3 cases.

Burns

Burns are a major problem in South Africa, resulting in 11 percent of injury-related deaths under age 15 years (see Fig. 18-1) and 17.5 percent of all trauma admissions to RXH in 1986 and 1987. This contrasts sharply with the United Kingdom, where in 1986, burns and scalds only constituted 5.2 percent of domestic injuries.[15]

Table 18-5 gives the rates for 3 population groups and shows that children under age 5 years are most at risk, as is the case in United States.[33] Rates for the White children compare well with developed and developing countries, but the rates for Coloureds are exceedingly high, especially under age 5 years. The burn death rates for Coloured children decreased from 1968 to 1979, coinciding with improved housing and facilities, but has been increasing slightly since 1979.

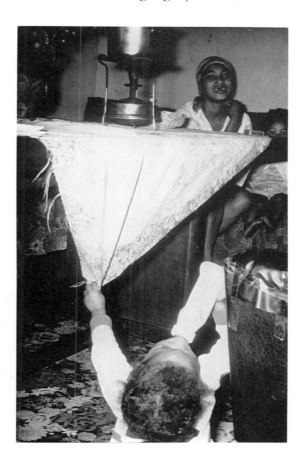

Figure 18-4. Typical mechanism of hot water scald from boiling water on primus stove

Eighty six percent of these deaths were fire burns[34] and the remainder were scalds, electrical, or chemical burns. This contrasts considerably with morbidity data, as 82 percent of all burn cases presenting to RXH and 71 percent requiring admission were scalds caused by hot water and other liquids. Over 90 percent of these affected less than 20 percent of the body surface area. Fire burns constituted only 13 percent of all burn admissions, but produced more serious injury in that they were responsible for 83 percent of deaths occurring in the RXH burn unit.[35] The majority of burn-injured children in the Cape Town area who require hospitalization are managed at RXH, where a Burn Unit is reserved for cases needing admission.

Of patients admitted in 1986 and 1987, 50 percent were less than 2 years old and 80 percent were under 5 years. In a 6 month prospective study of burned children admitted to RXH, de Wet and associates stressed the importance of overcrowding, particularly in the Black population, as a factor predisposing to burn injuries.[35] Food is cooked on primus stoves (kerosene fuel) and not infrequently on open fires. In their study, De Wet and colleagues calculated that 76 percent of all burns occurred indoors, of which 71 percent occurred in kitchens (Fig. 18-4). The most serious accidents occurred among squatters housed in make-shift shacks, where 70 percent of the burns proved fatal (Fig. 18-5). These data suggest that most burn injuries in local children are directly related to socioeconomic factors.

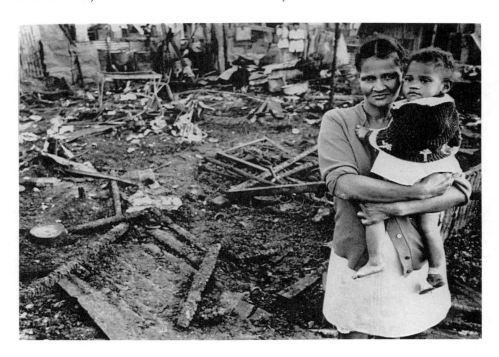

Figure 18-5. The aftermath of a shack fire (courtesy Willem Stassen, Die Burger Library)

Assaults: Homicide/abuse

Although assault accounted for only 6 percent of injury-related deaths under 15 years (see Fig. 18-1), there is a large group (14%) of deaths in which it was not determined if the injury was intentional or accidental, and in most of these the cause of injury was also undetermined. It is possible that a number of these cases are really assault/abuse, which would make assault a leading cause of death.

At RXH, assault/abuse represents only 3 percent of patients admitted for trauma and 2 percent of trauma outpatients. As in other countries the true incidence of child abuse in South Africa is unknown.[36,37] The annual increase in reported cases at the RXH in Cape Town (Fig. 18-6), especially those of child sexual abuse, has also been documented in Durban.[38] Hopefully, this reflects not only an increase in public awareness, but also the value of the multidisciplinary child protection teams that now exist in most metropolitan areas in South Africa.[37,38] Each team consists of consultant pediatricians or surgeons, clinical psychologists, and social workers. The latter liaise where necessary with regional child protection units of the South African Police and this system is aimed, so far successfully, at maximal detection of child abuse victims with a minimum of additional trauma to both child and family.

Between 1981 and 1985, firearm injuries accounted for 221 deaths in the group under age 15 years. Fifty four percent were the result of assault/homicide—some of these children being the victims of a spate of family slayings. From 1984 to 1987, 37 children under 15 were treated at the RXH trauma unit for firearm injuries, with a peak of 14 in 1985, coinciding with a period of civil unrest. These figures contrast with those in the United States, where firearm injuries are extremely high, and are,

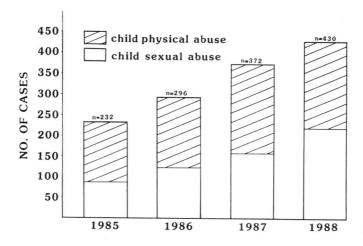

Figure 18-6. The increasing number of children with assault/abuse presenting at Red Cross Children's Hospital from 1985 to 1988

in fact, the second leading cause of injury deaths. Recent estimates indicate that 1,200 children die annually as a result of gunshot wounds and 800 more are injured in this manner—the majority of incidents being unintentional.[39]

Drowning

Drowning is the second most important cause of injury-related death in children in South Africa. The drowning death rates for 3 population groups are shown in Table 18-5. As in other countries, the age 1 to 4 year group is at greatest risk, and the rates for boys are almost always higher than those of girls, even under 1 year of age.

Despite the fact that Cape Town has high drowning rates,[40] immersion accounted for only 0.3 percent of the injuries seen at RXH during 1986 and 1987. Twenty seven were treated as out-patients, while 43 were admitted. A review of 107 patients admitted to RXH from 1976 to 1987, showed that 12 percent died and 7 percent of the survivors had neurological sequelae, which is in keeping with other hospital-based studies.[41] Total population studies from Hawaii and Australia have shown a far better outcome, with morbidity and mortality rates of under 5 percent.[42,43]

The sites of drowning accidents vary from one area of the country to another. Overall, 61 percent of children under age 15 years drown in dammed waters or rivers, 16.5 percent in swimming pools, 4.6 percent in baths or buckets, and only 3.2 percent in the ocean, while 14.7 percent drown in other sites (e.g., canals, lagoons, springs, holes, gutters, and in fact, any other container holding water).[44] In the White group, 61.6 percent drown in swimming pools, while 72.8 percent of the Black drowning deaths occur in dammed water or rivers.[44]

Forty six percent of the patients treated at RXH had been submerged in swimming pools and 18 percent in buckets—the latter incidents largely involving children of the Coloured and Black groups.[41] This high proportion of bucket immersions is unique in the medical literature,[40] and community-based studies are needed to determine if this finding is borne out in the community at large. Absence of running water in the home, overcrowding, and inadequate supervision of children are all causative factors.

Although Cape Town is a coastal city, only a small percentage of fatal and non-fatal immersion incidents in childhood occur in the ocean,[41] which is consistent with findings in Honolulu[43] and Brisbane,[41] and differs from the incidence in adult drowning.[40]

Poisoning

Poisoning is responsible for 4 percent of injury deaths, but represents considerable morbidity. The RXH has a Poisons Information Centre that provides advice on a 24-hour basis. In 1986 and 1987, a total of 2871 patients were seen at RXH for poisoning, and a further 2798 telephone calls were received. Twenty five percent of the cases were hospitalized as compared to the 9.5 percent admitted in 1967 to the Hospital for Sick Children, Toronto.[14]

As in other countries, the majority of cases (88.4%) involved children under age 5 years.[13,14] Medicines compose the largest group of poisoning sources and form 55 percent of admitted poisoning cases and 60 percent of out-patients. In sharp contrast to developed countries, 28 percent of RXH poisoning cases involve kerosene, which is the most commonly used domestic fuel in areas without electricity. It is used in stoves, lamps, heaters, and refrigerators. Local retailers sell kerosene in unlabelled wine and beverage bottles.[45] Although there has recently been a public awareness campaign (Fig. 18-7) to inform people of the danger, no

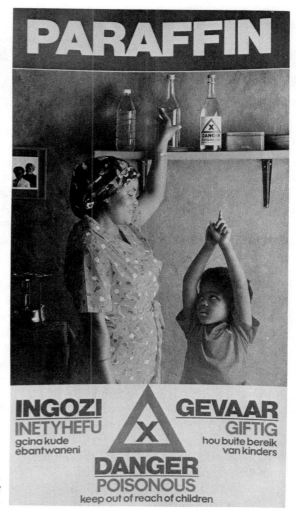

Figure 18-7. Poster used in a campaign to measure public awareness of paraffin poisoning and its dangers

legislation controls the sale of this poison in unsafe containers. In the United States, petroleum distillates have to be sold in child-resistant containers.[46]

Prevention

The magnitude of the childhood-injury problem is evident. Childhood injuries are not random events, occurring without pattern or predictability; their causes are foreseeable, researchable, and, to a great extent, avoidable. Unfortunately, these injuries are often referred to as "accidents," which allows them to be immediately interpreted as unavoidable incidents of chance or fate. They must be regarded as an epidemic and be given the same attention as other preventable diseases.[2] Local statistics are vital because it is futile to simply transplant preventative strategies that were developed in other countries and are based on their situations.

In 1978, the Child Safety Centre was established in the Department of Paediatric Surgery at the Institute of Child Health, University of Cape Town. Prior to this time, the Road Safety Council was the only body collecting road-injury statistics and producing public awareness campaigns in an attempt to reduce MVAs. For the first time, prospective collection of data was carried out, particularly with the opening of the Trauma Unit at the Red Cross War Memorial Children's Hospital. The statistics of injury-related deaths and morbidity are analysed and the incidence, type, and cause of childhood injuries evaluated. A study of the causes and nature of burns in childhood was started, in addition to an on-going project with the South African Bureau of Standards on fabric flammability.

Armed with these statistics, educational programs on prevention of some categories of injuries were complied, but problems with inadequate resources, and the linguistic and cultural differences among the various population groups had to be overcome. Despite these problems, the members of the Child Safety Centre have built a remarkable achievement record. The adult target groups reached include the nursing profession, workers in industry, social workers, medical students, and a wide variety of groups in the lay public. Community workers have been trained to teach safety awareness in their own communities. Excellent cooperation has been obtained from the Department of Education, with access being provided to school children and with various health groups.

The Child Safety Centre was instrumental in ensuring adequate specifications for type and installation of seat-belts and safety chairs for babies and children in motor vehicles, and is currently seeking legislative measures to protect children from the indiscriminate sale and dispensing of certain poisons, particularly kerosene. The National Road Safety Council is presently running an educational campaign, entitled, "The Child in Traffic Programme," which involves both school children and their parents.

The prevention of childhood injuries and research into the problem of injury are relatively new concepts in South Africa. However, a very real need exists for the pertinent information. In our mixed, complex society (with different trends existing within each ethnic group) there is an urgent need for the development of injury prevention programs that are culturally and socially appropriate. Community consultation is needed to achieve this. It is hoped that this will enable the formulation of more realistic education programs aimed at the various target groups. Similarly, this information will help in seeking and formulating legislative measures. As these programs proceed, it is also imperative that their effectiveness be constantly monitored and evaluated.

There are few areas of research in which the paucity of existing data relative to the scope of the problem shows such a wide discrepancy as with childhood injuries. The prevention of injuries remains low in the hierarchy of medical priorities, and progress in creating an awareness of the childhood injury problem with the South African public has been slow. Thus far, the role of the Child Safety Centre has been a pioneering one and can now be followed by a coordinated effort from the medical profession and other relevant disciplines, an effort designed to address the problem in a more scientific manner. A united front is required on a national basis because progress in injury prevention will be achieved only through the combined efforts of individuals, organizations, government, and community groups.

References

1. Central Statistical Services, Pretoria: Population Census 1985, Report No. 02-85-06, Human Sciences Research Council Estimates, 1985
2. Davis HF Jr, Schletty AV, Ing RT, Wiesner PJ: The 1990 objectives for the nation for injury prevention: A progress review. Publ Health Review 99:10, 1984
3. Burman S, Reynolds P (eds): Growing up in a divided society: The contexts of childhood in South Africa. In association with the Centre for Cross-cultural Research on Women, Queen Elizabeth House, Oxford University. Johannesburg, Raven Press, 1986
4. Smit P, Booysen JJ: Swart Verstedeliking: Proses, Patroon en Strategie. (Black Urbanization: Process, Pattern and Strategy). Cape Town, Tafelberg, 1981
5. Gulaid JA, Onwuachi-Saunders EC, Sacks JJ, Roberts D: Differences in death rates due to injury among Blacks and Whites, 1984. MMWR 37:25, 1988
6. Mare RD: Socio-economic effects on child mortality in the United States. Am J Pub Health 72:539, 1982
7. Vimpani G, Doudle M, Harris R: Child accident mortality in the Northern Territory, 1978–85. Med J Aust 148:392, 1988
8. Medical Research Council Technical Report No. 1, May 1987: Review of South African Mortality. 1984
9. Wyndham CH: Cause- and age-specific mortality rates from accidents, poisoning and violence. S Afr Med J 69:559, 1986
10. Taket A: Accident mortality in children, adolescents and young adults. World Health Stat Q 39:232, 1986
11. Knobel GJ, de Villiers JC, Parry CDH, Botha JL: The causes of non-natural deaths in children over a 15-year period in greater Cape Town. S Afr Med J 66:795, 1984
12. Colombani PM, Buck JR, Dudgeon DL et al: One-year experience in a regional paediatric trauma centre. J Ped Surg 20:8, 1985

13. Gallagher SS, Finison K, Guyer B, Goodenough S: The incidence of injuries among 87,000 Massachusetts children and adolescents. Am J Pub H 74:12, 1984
14. Shah CK: Epidemiology of injuries in childhood. In Finnegan S (ed): Care of the Injured Child, p 413. Baltimore, Williams and Wilkins, 1975
15. Dept of Trade and Industry (UK): Home accident surveillance system, 10th annual report, 1986
16. de Villiers JC, Jacobs M, Parry CDH, Botha JL: A retrospective study of head-injured children admitted to two hospitals in Cape Town. S Afr Med J 66:801, 1984
17. Rivara FP: Epidemiology of violent deaths in children and adolescents in the United States. Paediatrician 12:3, 1983–85
18. Institute of Biostatistics, Medical Research Council and Child Safety Centre, University of Cape Town: Unpublished data, 1989
19. Conn JM: Deaths from motor vehicle-related injuries, 1978–1984. MMWR 37(SS-1):5, 1988
20. McKellar A, Harte C: Head injuries in children and implications for their prevention (abstr). Annual International Congress of the British Association of Paediatric Surgeons, Athens, 1988
21. Central Statistical Services, Pretoria: Road Traffic Accidents Report, 1986
22. McDermott FT: Prevention of Road Accidents in Australia. Paediatrician 12:41, 1983–85
23. Peacock WJ: Editorial: Head injuries in children. S Afr Med J 66:789, 1984
24. Croft AW, Shaw DA, Cartlidge NEF: Head Injuries in Children. Br Med J 4:200, 1972
25. Brooke OG: Delayed effects of head injuries in children. Br Med J 296:948, 1988
26. Roux P: Pleural effusion following blunt chest injury in children. S Afr J Crit Care 4:21, 1988
27. Adler DD, Blane CE, Coran AG, Silver TM: Splenic trauma in the paediatric patient: The integrated roles of ultrasound and computed tomography. Paediatrics 78:576, 1986
28. Cywes S, Rode H, Millar AJW: Blunt liver trauma in children: Non-operative management. J Ped Surg 20:14, 1983
29. Editorial: Conservative management of the ruptured spleen. Lancet ii:777, 1988
30. Oldham KT, Guice KS, Ryckman F et al: Blunt liver injury in childhood: Evaluation of therapy and current perspective. Surgery 100:542, 1986
31. Bass DH, Mann MD, Cremin BJ: Unpublished data. A prospective comparison of computed tomography and radionuclide scan in the evaluation of liver and spleen injuries in children. 1989
32. Uthoff LB, Wyffels PL, Adams CS et al: A prospective study comparing nuclear scintigraphy and computerised axial tomography in the initial evaluation of the trauma patient. Ann Surg 198:611, 1983
33. Gulaid JA, Sattin RW, Waxweiler RJ: Deaths from residential fires 1978–84. MMWR 37(SS-1):39, 1988
34. Institute of Biostatistics, Medical Research Council and Child Safety Centre, University of Cape Town: Unpublished data, 1989
35. de Wet B, Davies MRQ, Cywes S: Die oorsake van brandwonde by kinders (The causes of burns in children). S Afr Med J 52: 969, 1977
36. Editorial: Implications of the Cleveland Inquiry. Br Med J 297:151, 1988
37. Kempe RS, Kempe CH: Sexual abuse of children and adolescents. New York, Freeman, 1984

38. Winship WS, Key JA, Damos ME, Jacob WAS: Examination of sexually abused children. S Afr Med J 71:437, 1987
39. Christoffel KK: American as apple pie: Guns in lives of US children and youth. Paediatrician 12:46, 1983–85
40. Davis S, Smith LS: The epidemiology of drowning in Cape Town 1980–83. S Afr Med J 68:739, 1985
41. Kibel SM, Nagel FO, Myers J, Cywes S: Childhood near drowning: A 12 year retrospective review. S Afr Med J (in press).
42. Pearn J: Neurological and psychometric studies in children surviving fresh water immersion accidents. Lancet 1:7, 1977
43. Pearn JH, Bart RD, Yamaoka R: Neurological sequelae after childhood near drowning: A total population study from Hawaii. Pediatrics 64:187, 1979
44. de Wet J: Unpublished report. An analysis of the drownings in South Africa of children 0–14 years for the year 1986
45. Rom S, van der Walt F, Leary P: Unpublished report. Memorandum on paraffin poisoning submitted to the Minister of Health, 1985

International Statistical Classification of Diseases and Causes of Death (I.C.D.) 1975, 9th revision
MAIN DISEASE GROUPS

Main Disease Groups	Classification
*Infectious and parasitic diseases	001–139
Neoplasms	140–239
*Endocrine, nutritional and metabolic diseases and immune disorders	240–279
Diseases of blood and blood-forming organs	280–289
Mental disorders	290–319
*Diseases of the nervous system and sense organs	320–389
Diseases of the circulatory system	390–459
*Diseases of the respiratory system	460–519
Diseases of the digestive system	520–579, 609 +
Diseases of the genitourinary system	580–629 (Excl.609 +)
Complications of pregnancy, childbirth and puerperium	630–676
Diseases of the skin and subcutaneous tissue	680–709
Diseases of the musculoskeletal system and connective tissue	710–739
*Congenital anomalies	740–759
*Certain conditions originating in the perinatal period	760–779
*Symptoms, signs and ill-defined conditions	780–799
*Accidents, poisoning and violence (external causes)	800–999

Note: * indicates the main cause groups in childhood shown in Table 18-1.
   + is an additional code used by Central Statistical Services, Pretoria

INDEX